CLASSICAL HOMEOPATHIC PRACTICE

A
SCIENTIFIC APPROACH

- *Case taking* • *Case processing* • *Miasmatic diagnosis*
- *Construction of totality* • *Repertorisation*
- *Simillimum* • *Potency selection*

Dr Anurag Deshmukh

Ex-Lecturer, Department of Case Taking and Homeopathic Repertory, Antarbharti Homeopathic Medical College, Nagpur, Maharashtra. Secretary, Homeopathic Study Circle, Nagpur, Maharashtra.

B. Jain Publishers (P) Ltd.
An ISO 9001 : 2000 Certified Company
USA—EUROPE—INDIA

CLASSICAL HOMEOPATHIC PRACTICE — A SCIENTIFIC APPROACH

First Edition: 2006
Second Revised Edition: 2010
1st Impression: 2010

All rights reserved. No part of this book may be reproduced, stored in a retrieval system or transmitted, in any form or by any means, mechanical, photocopying, recording or otherwise, without any prior written permission of the publisher.

© with the publisher

Published by Kuldeep Jain for
B. JAIN PUBLISHERS (P) LTD.
An ISO 9001 : 2000 Certified Company
1921/10, Chuna Mandi, Paharganj, New Delhi 110 055 (INDIA)
Tel.: 91-11-4567 1000 • Fax: 91-11-4567 1010
Email: info@bjain.com • Website: www.bjainbooks.com

Printed in India
J.J. Offset Printers

ISBN: 978-81-319-0940-9

*Dedicated to
my 'Guru'*
Dr S. Karnad
and my parents
Shri. G.G. Deshmukh
and
Smt. Radhika Deshmukh

Who will benefit from this book?

- A must read book for anybody interested in scientific study of homeopathic practice
- This book is for students of homeopathy in various universities, especially final year and post graduate students
- Interns aiming to practice homeopathy scientifically can also get acquainted to various aspects of homeopathic practice and repertorisation
- It is also intended to prove useful to teachers in homeopathic institutions
- Practitioners of all levels of experience can benefit from it
- Book that can serve as a guide in day-to-day clinical practice

FOREWORD

Homeopathic practice in its current form has far deviated from truth. Founded on the eternal law of cure - *Similia Similibus Curentur* and practiced for more than two centuries by homeopaths successfully on the basis of the cardinal principles that have evolved in its application. Today, its image is receiving a severe battering in the hands of none other than its own advocates. It is because the focus has totally shifted from the avowed mission of the practitioners to cure the sick to a more attractive object of making quick money. A glaring example of this is the flooding of market by thousands of pretentious products promising a cure for specific diseases throwing to winds in the process the time tested principles of individualisation and totality. Gone are those days of the stalwarts like Kent, Hering, Allen, Boger, and Roberts among others who sacrificed their lives to hold the truth alive through their unflinching adherence to the law of cure. Their devotion to science and to the cause of human suffering is history. The present genre of homeopaths, the hippocrates that they are, only swear by their name but, when it comes to commercial propositions, sweep under the carpet the rich heritage of knowledge they have left.

To a young entrant to homeopathy there is a perpetual conflict to choose between the values that have been thrust down his throat as a student in the class of *Organon of Medicine*, by his teachers and the diametrically opposite soft option of prescribing patents in his practice when he leaves the institution. Inevitably, the attraction is towards the path of least resistance.

To the few desirous to stay with the science and to know the rational art of healing the road is long and winding. Their quest for knowledge appears a distant dream.

In his work, the author has articulated his own experiences and the pangs of agony he went through in getting an insight into the scientific method of healing. If his experience serves to open the eyes of other budding homeopaths entering the field the object of this work is best accomplished.

I wish him success.

January 12, 2005 **Dr S. Karnad**
Nagpur *Ex-Member,*
India *Board of Studies in Homeopathy,*
Nagpur University.
Ex-Director, Institute of Clinical Research, Nagpur.
Founder President, Homeopathic Study Circle, Nagpur.

FOREWORD

World of homeopathic practice today lies in a total chaos. Clashes between various schools and approaches within homeopathy have further worsened the situation. The obvious reason for that seems to be the difference in interpretation of the Organon and other philosophical texts, the difference in understanding the practical implications of the terms and concepts present in these texts and consequently failure in application. Homeopathy is an applied science and the changes observed in the homeopathic field over all these years are rather disturbing, especially when it comes to application of principles to practice.

'Classical Homeopathic Practice — A Scientific Approach' by Dr Anurag Deshmukh is a noble and appreciable attempt and a need of the hour. Abstract of particular topics given in blocks reflects good presentation. Chapter No. 15, The 20 Don'ts of Homeopathic Practice, is very important for every homeopath.

This book is strongly recommended for publication.

Dr Mridula Pandey

PREFACE TO THE SECOND EDITION

The tremendous response to the first edition of this work suggests that the book was able to address the need of guidance in clinical practice. I have received many phone calls and mails, informing me that this work has proved to be a worthy edition to the homeopathic profession in general and homeopathic literature in particular.

A word of thanks is due to all the homeopathic practitioners, lecturers and students who have accepted the approach and appreciated the guidelines for practice incorporated in this work.

I thank Mr Kuldeep Jain of B. Jain Publishers Pvt. Ltd. and Dr Mridula Pandey for the encouragement and keen interest shown in bringing out the revised and enlarged second edition.

The necessary corrections have been made. Illustrative cases have been added in order to demonstrate the application of homeopathic philosophy and the various methods and techniques incorporated in the work. Keeping in mind the difficulties faced by practitioners in getting the 'Mentals' a new chapter on 'Knowing Patient's Psyche' has been added which is hoped to further enhance the utility of the book for everyone.

I hope that the readers would find the second edition of 'Classical Homeopathic Practice- A Scientific Approach' invaluable and more useful throughout the arduous but incredibly rewarding journey of homeopathic practice.

Anurag Deshmukh
Nagpur, India
dradeshmukhin@yahoo.co.in

PREFACE TO THE FIRST EDITION

Any system of medicine can be called an effective system of treating diseases only on the basis of the efficiency of its followers, the people who profess and practice it. As the victory of the team depends upon the quality of players, similarly, the quality or efficacy of a 'pathy' depends upon the efficiency and quality of its 'practitioners.' Efficiency and quality in turn depends on the successful application of laws, which in case of homeopathy is the law of similars.

Homeopathy is an applied science but the changes observed in the homeopathic field over all these years are rather disturbing, especially when it comes to application of principles to practice. Misinterpretation and total inability to comprehend the 'practical implications of homeopathic philosophy' and lack of scientific approach to practice together with the commercialization of physicians and pharmacists has led to the production of large number of, what I call 'Pseudo-homeopaths', the pathological prescribers and combination prescribers. Capacity to pull large number of patients rather than providing quality treatment has become the measure of a physician's efficiency. Homeopathic medical education has unfortunately failed to produce high quality homeopathic physicians who can put in to practice what they had learnt as a student. Hahnemann, Kent, Boenninghausen, Hering, Boger and numerous other names in the galaxy of homeopathic heroes inspire many to be like them, but in most of the cases, they miserably fail when it comes to actual homeopathic practice. Why? What goes wrong? Answer is obvious; we have failed to bring homeopathic practice to classrooms. Homeopathic students today feel insecure and unmotivated inspite of more than five years of training at graduation level, which hardly makes them capable to handle all types of cases. The inability of some teachers in making students understand the practical aspect of homeopathy has also contributed to the miseries of homeopathy.

World of homeopathic practice today lies in total chaos, as all the phenomenon described above has given rise to different sections of homeopaths practicing homeopathy in their own way, with some of them practicing in a very bizarre way. Clashes between various 'schools' and approaches within homeopathy have further worsened the situation. The obvious reason for that seems to be the difference in interpretation of the Organon of Medicine and other philosophical texts, the difference in understanding the practical implications of the terms and concepts contained in these texts and consequently failure in application. We have failed to apply philosophy to practice; we are drifting away from Hahnemann's teachings. Consequently the number of true Hahnemannian homeopaths left in the field can be counted on the fingertips. This is because although we know that homeopathic philosophy and homeopathic practice are two sides of the same coin and cannot be separated but, in actual practice, we divide them into separate compartments as we are seldom taught how to translate philosophical laws in to practice. All these observations during my association with homeopathy as a student, as a physician and now as a teacher led me to think of presenting a work to the profession that would emphasize and explain the practical implications of the various concepts in homeopathic philosophy.

This book is not intended to be a textbook, but would be of great help to the students and the beginners in practice, in understanding 'what homeopathic practice is all about' and getting oriented to it. This book discusses the implementational aspects of homeopathic practice. Through this book I have tried to demonstrate the application of homeopathic principles to practice. The chapter on homeopathic physician will make the reader, especially fresh homeopathic graduate, aware of the attitude and the type of clinical training necessary for scientific homeopathic practice and the qualities that need to be cultivated if he wishes to be a successful (Hahnemannian) homeopath. It will also introduce him to various means of acquiring clinical knowledge. How to conduct case taking? This is a frequently asked question. Therefore, chapter on case taking deals with practical aspect of case taking, and is full of practical tips and hints. Case processing is another important part of homeopathic practice and I have tried to simplify the complexities involved in it. Clinical implications of the concept of totality have been focused upon in the chapter on totality. Choice of the right remedy is one of the most perplexing dilemmas, especially for a neophyte and hence it has been addressed in as clear terms as possible in the related chapter. The matter of *Potency Selection* has been dealt with scant attention in most of the homeopathic literature till now. As a result many students and beginners are in total dark with regards to various factors that need to be considered while selecting potency for any given case. I have tried to explain the basic principles and the various criteria on which potency selection should be done if one wishes to have a scientific basis to his potency selection. All the teachings in homeopathy focus mainly on what should be done but what should not be done in homeopathic practice is seldom taught; considering this fact, I have also dealt with the don'ts of homeopathic practice in one of the chapters. I have tried to make the subject as transparent and as comprehensive as possible. In spite of the rich and varied homeopathic literature, as a student I always felt the need for something more than classroom talks, something which would give me practical hints for practicing homeopathy and applying its principles. This book is my small endeavor directed towards this end.

A book is no replacement for the experience which is the best teacher as far as practicing homeopathy is concerned, but I would feel rewarded if the book is able to fulfill, at least up to some extent, the long felt need of practical guidance in homeopathic practice. I hope it will serve as a bridge to the continuously increasing gap between theory and practice.

I am blessed to have been guided by my guru Dr S. Karnad who taught me through clinical study, an 'applied homeopathic philosophy' and helped me in my efforts to become a ' Scientific Prescriber'. Without his teachings I would not have been in a position to even think of creating any such work. I also acknowledge the help I received from my brother Dr Rashmin Deshmukh who took the pains of going through the manuscript and offered valuable suggestions. My parents and my wife Tanisha were a great source of encouragement when I was working on the book. I would also like to put on record my sincere gratitude to my students who inspired and motivated me to undertake this work.

I cannot claim this work to be perfect and would humbly welcome all your impressions, comments and suggestions about this effort.

March 6, 2005 **Anurag Deshmukh**
92, Mandar Apartments,
Pandey Layout, Khamla,
Nagpur 440025 (India)
Ph.: (0712)2283935
Email: dradeshmukhin@yahoo.co.in

ABOUT THE AUTHOR

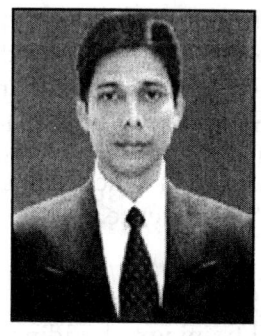

Dr Anurag Deshmukh was born on 8 June, 1972 at New Delhi. Author's parents were keenly interested in study of Homeopathy and used to prescribe homeopathic remedies to acquaintances and relatives for day-to-day ailments. Thus, born in an environment conducive to homeopathy, he was inclined to opt for homeopathy as his career. He completed his studies in homeopathy from Ahmednagar Homoeopathic Medical College, Ahmednagar in the year 1993. As a student he was among the toppers in both academic accomplishments as well as extra curricular activities.

With a view to gain wide experience in Homeopathic practice he worked with various reputed homeopaths. He also had the privilege of working as an assistant physician with Dr S. Karnad, a legendary figure in homeopathy in India. After developing his skills in classical homeopathy, he has been devoted to fulltime homeopathic practice since more than a decade and has a wide experience of treating complicated cases with classical homeopathy.

He functioned as the lecturer and incharge of department of Case taking and Homeopathic Repertory in Antarbharti Homoeopathic Medical College and Hospital, Dabha, Nagpur during the years 2001 and 2002. He is not only a strong advocate of practicing homeopathy in accordance with the principles and philosophy of homeopathy but is also uncompromising wherever principles are involved. His affection for students prompted him to create a work that would bridge the gap between theory and practice, the need for which is usually felt by fresh graduates, as a result, this book was born. The book is an expression of his strong desire and zeal to propagate a scientific approach to Homeopathic practice.

He has delivered talks and given case presentations on wide ranging topics in both local and national level seminars and conferences. Recently he had the privilege of guiding the participants at the P.G.workshop on 'Selecting the Simillimum' which was appreciated due to its 'case-centered' approach. His seminars are always full of practical tips and hints which make them more practical and interesting for the audience.

He is currently the Hon. Director of *'Systematic Homoeopathic Practice Orientation and Training Programme.'*(SHOT) Nagpur, India. This programme aimed at giving practical training to budding homeopaths, was designed by him in the year 2005. Since then, inspite of his preoccupation with busy practice he finds time to provide guidance to interns and fresh homeopathic graduates who face numerous difficulties while practicing homeopathy. He is also the Jt. Secretary, Homoeopathic Study Circle (HSC) and takes active interest in organizing academic discussions under the aegis of HSC established in 1965 (one of the oldest organizations of homeopathic physicians in central India). He had organized the Scientific Seminar in April 2002 at Nagpur, as part of the Hahnemann birth anniversary celebrations. The seminar got an overwhelming response from Homeopathic fraternity from all over Vidarbha. He is also a resource person and Hon. Advisor to Orange City Homoeopaths Association, Nagpur.

Besides, he is a freelance writer and has to his credit many articles on homeopathy and other subjects which have been published in prominent newspapers and magazines of English as well as vernacular languages.

CONTENTS

Dedication... *iii*
Who will benefit from this book .... *iv*
Foreword... *v*
Foreword... *vii*
Preface to the Second Edition .... *ix*
Preface to the First Edition .... *xii*
About the Author .... *xv*

Chapter 1

Introduction to Homeopathic Practice....................3
    Homeopathic Practice: An Overview 3
    What is Homeopathic Practice?.................................7
    Components of Homeopathic Practice 7
        The Homeopath 7
        The Patient..9
    Clinical Procedures in Homeopathic Practice 11
        Clinical Interview (Case taking) 11
        Clinical Diagnosis..12
        Case Processing 13
        Miasmatic Diagnosis 13
        Construction of Totality 14
        Repertorisation Procedure 14
        Selection of Single Remedy 14
        Potency Selection 15
        Planning and Programming of Treatment 15

Chapter 2

The Clinical Setup 19
    Financial Resources 20

Location / Site of Clinic 22
    An Ideal Location 22
Interiors of the Clinic 25
    Lighting 25
    Storage 26
    Furniture 27
    Equipments 28
    Decor 28
Clinical Timings 30
Fee Structure 32
Physician's Attire 33

Chapter 3
Homeopathic Physician - Redefined 37

Chapter 4
Secrets of Effective Case-taking 51
Introduction 51
Difficulties in Conducting Inquiry 53
    Obstacles due to Patient 53
    Obstacles due to Physician Himself 56
Before the Clinical Session 58
Art of Communication 60
Establishing 'Rapport' and Skilled Listening 61
    Tips for Rapport Building & Effective
    Communication 65
Five Key Aspects of Clinical Interview 66
    The Consulting Room / Chamber 67
    Physician's Attitude and Behaviour 68
    Listening 70
    Questioning 71
    Recording 73
Inquiry in Paediatric Cases 74

Observation and Examination of Children 74
Physical Examination 78
Documentation in Homeopathic Practice 80
Proforma of Case taking................................ 83
Appendix A 84
Appendix B 93
Appendix C 93

Chapter 5

Knowing Patient's 'Psyche': A Systematic Approach ... 97

The mental state 99
Prerequisites for perceiving mental state 101
What to ask? 101
Interpreting patient's story 104
Illustrative case I 107
Illustrative case II 117
A case for working 131

Chapter 6

Clinical Diagnosis 139

Value of Diagnosis 140
Steps in Diagnosis 144
    Interpretation of Clinical Features 144
    Physical Examination 147
    Investigations 148
    Differential Diagnosis 149

Chapter 7

Integrated Approach to Case Processing 153

Concept of Analysis 155
Types of Symptoms 157
    Common symptoms 158

      Uncommon and Characteristic Symptoms 160
      Generals 164
            Mental Generals 165
            Physical Generals 166
            Negative Generals 167
            Pathological Generals 168
            Concomitant Generals 168
      Particulars 169
      Concept of Evaluation in Practice 170
      Synthesis of Case 172

Chapter 8

The Art of Perceiving 'Totality' 177
      What is Totality? 177
      What is Patient's Image or 'Portrait'? 178
      Totality - A 'Homeopathic Diagnosis' 179
      Prerequisites for Perceiving Totality 180
      Clinical Implications 181
      Method of Erecting Totality 183
      Tips for Clinical Judgement of Totality 187
      Illustrative Case 188

Chapter 9

Scientific Approach to Repertorisation 201
      Selection of Repertory for a Case 205
      Symptom to Rubric Translation 207
      Construction of Repertorial Syndrome (RS) 207
      Choice of Eliminating Symptom 209
      Use of Cross-Repertorisation 210
      Appendix D 212
      Illustrative Case 213

Chapter 10

Working Methods of Repertorisation 227

Methods in General 227
    Thumb-finger Method 228
    Old Method or Plain Paper Method 228
    Modern Method or Repertorial Sheet Method ... 229
    Mechanical Method 229
    Eliminating Method 231
    Total Addition Process 232
Methods According to Philosophical Background 232
    Hahnemann and Boenninghausen's Method 233
    Kent's Method 233
    Working on Physical Generals 233
    Working on Peculiarity 233
    Working on Pathological Changes 233
    Working on Technical Nosology 234

Chapter 11

How to Select the Right Remedy? 237
    Right Thinking for Right Selection 240
    Establishing Similarity 243
    Criteria for Establishing Similarity 245
    Self-assessment 246
    Techniques of Prescribing 247
        Acute Prescribing 249
        Chronic Prescribing 252
    Inference 253

Chapter 12

Miasmatic Diagnosis 257
    Evolution of Miasmatic Theory 258
    Scientific Foundations of Miasmatic Theory 261
    Miasmatic Diagnosis 262
        Definition 262
        Need for Miasmatic Diagnosis 264

Comparative Table of Miasms 266
Table of Miasms 267

Chapter 13
Fundamentals of Potency Selection 275
Evolution of Theory of 'Small Dose' and 'Potency' .. 275
Susceptibility and 'Susceptibility-Potency'
Interrelationship 279
    Internal Environment 280
    External Environment 280
Laws of Potency Selection 284
Potency Types in Centesimal Scale 285
Scientific Basis of Potency Selection 285
    Onset of Disease 286
    Nature of Pathology 287
    Type of Symptoms 287
    Nature of Selected Remedy 287
    Constitution 288
    Age 288
    Sex 288
    Occupation 289
    Past History 289

Chapter 14
Skills of Successful Case Management 293
Remedy Administration 295
    Managing Remedy Stock 295
    Method of Remedy Administration 296
    Time of Remedy Administration 298
Dietary Recommendations 299
Repetition Strategy 301
Scheduling Follow-ups 303
Follow-up Prescription 304

    Recording Patient's Responses 305
    Interpretation of Patient's Responses 307
    Placebo Prescribing 313

Chapter 15
The 20 Don'ts of Homeopathic Practice 319

Chapter 16
Clinical Training in Homeopathic Practice 325
    Institute of Clinical Research 327
    Athenian School of Homeopathic Medicine 328
    Clinical Training Center for Classical Homeopathy ... 329
    Systematic Homoeopathic Practice Orientation and
    Training Programme (SHOT) 330
    Homoeopathic Study Circle 331
    Dr Robin Murphy, ND 332
    Dr Frederik Schroyens, MD 333
    Dr Roger van Zandvoort 334
    Dr Luc De Schepper, MD 335
    Dr Jeremy Sherr 335

Homeopathy on Internet 337
    Bibliography 339

CHAPTER I

Introduction to Homeopathic Practice

- ❖ Homeopathic Practice: An Overview — 3
- ❖ What is Homeopathic Practice? — 7
- ❖ Components of Homeopathic Practice — 7
  - The Homeopath — 7
  - The Patient — 9
- ❖ Clinical Procedures in Homeopathic Practice — 11

CHAPTER I

INTRODUCTION TO HOMEOPATHIC PRACTICE

HOMEOPATHIC PRACTICE: AN OVERVIEW

Medicine today covers a vast field. It has varied specialized branches. It is split into different disciplines in order to learn and teach it. Homeopathy can also be regarded as a specialized branch of medicine. The medical field in general has undergone remarkable changes in the last 50 years. There has been a steady rise in the cost of treatment and medicines.

The rising drug costs, the side effects of medicines (allopathic) plus the inability to get permanent cure have all contributed in bringing to fore the disadvantages of the modern medicine. All this has led to recognition of homeopathy as a good alternative. In many of the Asian countries, homeopathy is being more and more appreciated. There has been a gradual realization of the fact that homeopathy has multiple benefits. All this has led to the fact that homeopathy is no more viewed as just an 'alternative therapy.' It is beginning to be regarded as a specialized branch of medical science.

India, Pakistan and Bangladesh are the countries where homeopathy is more popular. Amongst them, India has the largest number of homeopaths. India is the only country which has officially recognized homeopathy as a system of medicine legally at par with all other systems of medicine including allopathy. There are over 140 government recognized homeopathic medical colleges in the country. Nowhere in the world does the homeopathic system enjoys such privileges and opportunities as in India.

Inspite of this few of the colleges are producing homeopaths of the right standard because majority of the institutions have extremely poor teaching equipment. Very few have an indoor hospital and most of the beds remain empty due to inefficiency of attending and visiting physicians and also due to financial stringency of management. A fresh homeopath therefore is not fully aware of what homeopathic practice is all about.

Even if he knows a little about practice it is because of his personal efforts. A homeopathic student seldom receives practical training (in true sense) with regards to homeopathic practice. Our educational institutions do not take any pains in training students in clinical homeopathy. Homeopathic educational institutions go on producing homeopathic degree holders or graduates but fail in producing 'homeopaths.'

The result is disastrous. 'Rapid, rough and permanent destruction of health' is what today's injudicious homeopathic practice is causing to the patients. It is exactly contrast of what Hahnemann wanted homeopathic practice to deliver (Rapid, gentle and permanent restoration of health).

Innumerable personal theories and bizarre methods of prescription making dominate the scene of homeopathic practice. There is no standardization of methods of homeopathic practice. Homeopathic practice today is nothing more than prescribing and dispensing anything labeled as "homeopathic" without knowing why and how it acts? Physicians prescribe without even bothering for a second whether it is indicated in a particular case or not? It is observed that for some inexplicable reasons, homeopaths take on cases where they cannot deliver. Due to lack of competence and inability to understand limitations of homeopathic system, they go on treating patients without the desired results. It is rare to find a homeopathic general practice based on principles. A very small number of homeopaths care about maintaining case records. Still fewer make an attempt to arrive at reasonable clinical diagnosis. There is dearth of practitioners who succeed in effecting cures in the true Hahnemannian sense.

Qualified medical practitioners of other systems of medicine and laypersons practicing homeopathy have made the situation miserable. The number of people practicing homeopathy has increased by leaps and bounds but the quality of practice has equally deteriorated. Successful homeopathic practice today means successful from monetary point of view.

Since past few years there is an increase in the number of people aware of the benefits of homeopathy. Many people visit a homeopath hoping to get relief and cure without side effects. When they do not get the expected relief they conclude that homeopathy is ineffective and has failed. They do not realize that it is the homeopath who has failed and not homeopathy. This is because they don't know what is homeopathy. They have no idea with regards to what constitutes right type of homeopathy. This needs consumer education and quality control. These issues still remain unaddressed. A very small number of homeopaths take pains to educate the patient, so that he knows what is right and what is wrong.

Large majority of homeopaths do not receive proper training. Therefore, they find it difficult to practice homeopathy according to its basic principles. A large majority employs methods which are contrary to principles and logic of homeopathy. Since Hahnemann's time there have been spurious physicians who brought disgrace to homeopathy. Even Hahnemann criticized them and was surprised as to how these so called homeopaths disposed large number of patients everyday. The situation remains same even today. Dr. Dhawale very vividly describes the current scenario. He states, "we have just to walk in to any well-attended charitable dispensary with the signboard 'homeopathic' to discover a large number of patients being processed through the mill. All appear to be happy, so many people are receiving 'homeopathic treatment' and they would not be coming in such large numbers were they not be benefiting." So the logic runs! The numbers become the criteria of judgment. Do we assess the clinical records and evaluate them for the quality of care delivered?

The same picture is obtained in our hospitals attached to the medical colleges. The standard of the leading institutes and private homeopathic practice is presenting a gloomy picture. Allen aptly remarks, "As our institutions are so are our people."

The scene is extremely chaotic. If we want order out of chaos, we must train budding homeopaths with regards to the methods and techniques of practicing homeopathy scientifically. If we want our methods to be of right type they should be based on philosophy and guided by principles. If homeopathic practice is to progress in true sense then we must come out of compartmentalization of homeopathic education in to various disconnected subjects like Organon, Materia Medica, Repertory and Practice of Medicine.

The present day formal homeopathic education treats these subjects as watertight compartments. There is complete lack of integration. An integrated multidisciplinary approach to homeopathy in both learning and practice can only lead to production of efficient and scientific homeopaths. This only can improve the quality of homeopathic practice and bring it out of its present day pathetic condition. Principles cannot be translated into practice unless efficient techniques are evolved. Right methodology and technique for rational homeopathic practice can be developed through principle based, logical, integrated approach to homeopathy. The subsequent chapters of the book explain and define the methods and techniques of homeopathic practice. These methods are based on homeopathic principles and logic. It is aimed to guide the practitioners and students in practicing homeopathy scientifically. The book is aimed to make the budding homeopaths well oriented and better equipped to begin his/her private practice. One is sure to get better and rapid results in various types of cases if one follows the guidelines in the book.

WHAT IS HOMEOPATHIC PRACTICE?

Homeopathic practice can be defined as the art of applying the science and logic of homeopathy while taking the case, prescribing for the actual patient, understanding, assessing and analyzing the results and following through the subsequent prescriptions to cure. Successful homeopathic practice represents a scientific application of the fundamental principles of homeopathy to an individual instance of disease.

COMPONENTS OF HOMEOPATHIC PRACTICE

Homeopath and the patient are the two important components of homeopathic practice. One should be fully aware of the role each one plays and various related aspects that govern them.

THE HOMEOPATH

The success in homeopathic practice depends greatly upon the one who is practicing it i.e. the homeopathic physician. He is the master of the show. To be a good physician one must be a good human being first. To be an efficient homeopath *(read chapter 3 also)* one must possess various areas of knowledge. The knowledge includes command of basic facts about medical science in general and homeopathy in particular. A homeopath must have a sound knowledge of medicine, homeopathic philosophy, materia medica and repertory. He should be in a position to determine obstacles to recovery and cure so that they are dealt with effectively.

Only knowledge is not sufficient to make him an efficient homeopath. He should have good communication skills and qualities like patience, persistence and philosophical bent of mind. Determination and commitment to homeopathy also plays a part in making of a homeopath. The knowledge and skills acquired by a homeopath during his student life makes the job of practicing homeopathy easier for him. He would have fewer problems in managing his patients if he has mastered the art of clinical as well as therapeutic diagnosis.

A homeopath has to perform various duties for efficient patient management. The manifold duties of a homeopath are summarised by Dr. Elizabeth Wright Hubbard. She states that, our duty to them as homeopaths is manifold:

First in importance, is to pick the right remedy and to remove obstacles to cure.

- To stop harmful practices and give placebo if needed to keep them from taking other things.
- To give them enough understanding of homeopathic philosophy to co-operate in their cure.
- To institute proper diet, hygiene, protection and state of mind.

Second, to win the patient's confidence by what you are—by your profound humanity, by your ability to see them as they could be, whole.

- By your painstaking thoroughness in questioning and in examination.

Introduction to Homeopathic Practice

- By your attitude towards science, having tests when these are harmless and diagnostically helpful.

During the course of homeopathic practice a homeopath may be required to play various roles such as a psychiatrist, a diagnostician, a hygienist, and a pediatrician etc. But a homeopath must recognize his personal and technical limitations. He should not hesitate to take services of other physicians (e.g. pathologist, radiologist, endocrinologist etc.) who are specially qualified in a particular branch of medical science. A wise physician always keeps in mind what is good for his patient and pathy.

THE PATIENT

The patient has high expectations from a homeopath because more often than not he visits a homeopath when the modern system of medicine has failed to satisfy him. He is full of worries regarding curability of his ailments. Majority of times he expects miracles from a homeopath. Usually such patients come with a large heap of laboratory investigations, X-rays and other tests carried out by earlier physicians. Here the homeopath must not get overzealous and over enthusiastic. He should avoid making tall claims and false promises. A rational homeopath must first diagnose the disease and see the extent of pathological changes in the patient. After this he is in a better position to decide and inform the patient what he can do and how much progress to expect. If the homeopath feels that the case is beyond the realms of homeopathy, he should not hesitate to reject the case and refer it to some physician of other system of medicine. This would reduce the number of failures of the homeopath as well as homeopathy.

One may get a large variety of patients in practice. The behavioural pattern varies from patient to patient. Some are violent, arrogant, manipulative while some do not cooperate while conducting the clinical interview. Such patients predispose the physician to error. The best way to handle them is to be calm, composed and firm at times. The physician should avoid getting anxious and angry when he gets a problem patient. Considerable amount of patience and poise is demanded in handling such patients. Physician should find out the cause of patient's abnormal behaviour and do what he can to make the patient comfortable. Physician should listen to patient's concerns and try to reassure him.

Majority of times patients who are fed up with their illness behave arrogantly. They may behave abnormally due to their bad experience with the earlier physician. A homeopath should therefore never forget that besides cure a patient expects the physician to listen to him. He expects the physician to be gentle, caring, compassionate, and non-judgmental. He wants a doctor who informs him about the nature of disease he is suffering from and the future of his illness. Besides, he also expects his physician to be a competent homeopath having knowledge of recent advances in medical science.

Homeopathy is very demanding with respect to both the homeopath and the patient. A patient has to be a good observer of his own systems, otherwise the homeopath is most likely to fail due to lack of characteristics in the case. The patients who have previously taken homeopathic treatment from a good homeopath report their symptoms well. The cases where the patients know little about homeopathy, they need to be educated by the physician regarding certain technical aspects of homeopathic practice. The physician should indicate the type of information necessary for homeopathic treatment. Initially some patients may not be ready to furnish detailed information as they think it is unnecessary. The physician should have the ability to convince such patients. Physician should convey the reasons behind the necessity of recording minute details and accurate observations. If the patient hides facts then the physician would never be able to give results.

To be a successful homeopath one must always try to establish a good personal relationship that encourages the patient to confide in him.

CLINICAL PROCEDURES IN HOMEOPATHIC PRACTICE

In Hahnemann's Organon and homeopathic philosophy we find very practical advice regarding the actual clinical procedures that need to be carried out while treating a patient in homeopathic practice. A physician who wants his practice to be scientific and meaningful must be fully aware of all the procedures involved. The homeopathic clinical procedures demand great deal of effort and hard work on the part of the treating physician. These procedures help in translating philosophy into practice, which is, must for getting results with homeopathy. Various scientific procedures involved in homeopathic practice (details of each are given in subsequent chapters of the book) can be listed as follows:

1. Clinical Interview (Case taking including physical examination and laboratory investigations)
2. Clinical Diagnosis
3. Case Processing
4. Miasmatic Diagnosis
5. Construction of Totality
6. Repertorization Procedure
7. Selection of Single Remedy (Simillimum)
8. Potency Selection
9. Planning and Programming of Treatment

1. CLINICAL INTERVIEW (CASE TAKING)

Clinical interview is the backbone of a scientific homeopathic practice. A homeopath without a well-taken case is like a batsman without a bat. Accuracy in prescription making largely depends on good case taking. A homeopath cannot afford to be weak in this very important area of homeopathic practice. A physician, who does not have sufficient evidence to make a satisfactory prescription, often loses his patient, as there are no results or partial results. Besides, a well-taken case on paper is a proof of the work done by physician. It helps a great deal in proving homeopathy as a scientific system of medicine, once the results are obtained. Every homeopath must strive to develop his skills of case taking right from the beginning of his career. Various books on the subject may help a homeopath but the best way to acquire the skills of case taking is repeated exposure to it. Every new case taken adds something to physician's investigative skills. A physician's experience should be calculated by the number of well-taken and well-treated cases, not by the number of years spent in the field.

It requires:
- Unprejudiced obervation.
- Perception.
- Efficient communication.

One must not forget that case taking is not merely a question-answer session based on a predetermined format. Case taking involves observation (*unprejudiced observation*), perception and efficient communication. In cases where due to some reason patient is unable to convey his complaints by speech, observation becomes the only means of taking a case. A homeopath must be skilled in getting the required information especially in cases where the linguistic deficiency of the patient and his attendants hamper the case taking. Proficiency in homeopathic practice is almost always the result of a well-taken case.

2. CLINICAL DIAGNOSIS

A homeopath's prescription is based on the totality of symptoms, therefore he can prescribe even before the diagnosis is done. Homeopathy has this distinct advantage. But this facility to prescribe on symptoms has given rise to the most popular misconception that diagnosis is not necessary for a homeopath and pathological tests are also unwanted. Unfortunately even today many homeopaths under this misconception prescribe indiscriminately without any consideration to nature of disease and the extent of pathology. This attitude has proved damaging for both physician and the science of homeopathy. The knowledge of diagnosis enables the physician to choose his cases. It enables him to eliminate cases where the extent of pathology makes it necessary to apply surgical or other measures. Diagnosis has various other advantages too. The reader is requested to read the chapter on clinical diagnosis where this topic is discussed in greater detail.

3. CASE PROCESSING

The large amount of data collected during clinical interview is confusing and useless, unless it is processed. Case processing consists of analysis (classification), evaluation and synthesis. It converts the large mass of symptoms in to a meaningful totality and it is therefore very important in making a prescription. Case processing serves as a filter that eliminates unwanted material in the case. Case processing makes the job of establishing individuality easier for the homeopathic physician.

4. MIASMATIC DIAGNOSIS

A homeopath has to determine the predominant miasm in the case, because the remedy selected should be similar at the level of miasmatic expression too. Similarity at other levels without similarity at the miasmatic level would be a partial similarity. A physician who ignores this fact often fails to cure his patients. Although the subject of miasms is still debated, one should not ignore this aspect in a scientific clinical practice. Relapses of chronic complaints are inevitable unless the miasm in the background is remedied.

5. CONSTRUCTION OF TOTALITY

The heart and the art of homeopathic practice lie in the perception of patient's totality. Totality is logically arranged syndrome of characteristics, which forms the image of the patient, so that a suitable remedy resembling it can be selected. The concept of totality is the essence of homeopathic system of medicine. It is proved since the time of Hahnemann that a totality based prescription never fails. Physician's success in treating patients with homeopathic remedies is directly proportional to the successful application of the concept of totality.

6. REPERTORISATION PROCEDURE

Repertorization is often labeled as a laborious and time-consuming part of homeopathy by majority of homeopaths. Many therefore avoid it. Repertorization is very useful in complicated cases as it narrows down the indicated remedies.

Repertorization procedure can prove disastrous for the case if carried out mechanically. Selection of rubrics must be carefully done. One must not forget that repertory gives back what we feed to it. If we expect the repertory to deliver quality then we must also have a qualitative approach towards the selection of rubrics for repertorization. The right approach to repertorization procedure is explained in detail in subsequent chapters of the book.

7. SELECTION OF SINGLE REMEDY

Only a single remedy is similar to a given case at any point of time. Remedy selection can be called as the 'art' part of homeopathic practice. The remedy selected should have similarity with the patient at various levels. Similarity at the level of mind and body (characteristics), similarity at the level of miasmatic background and similarity at the level of functional and structural changes. Only a prescription that satisfies all these conditions is 'homeopathic' in true sense. At times remedy selection becomes

Introduction to Homeopathic Practice 15

difficult even for an experienced homeopath. The solution lies in the knowledge of criteria and logic of remedy selection. Remedy selection is theoretically simple to understand but difficult to implement hence the logic and techniques of remedy selection are dealt with in detail in this book.

8. POTENCY SELECTION

Similarity at the level of potency is equally essential otherwise the results are unsatisfactory and may be delayed. The question of potency is the most debated one as different sections of homeopaths have different opinions and views regarding potency selection. The methods of potency selection are also as varied as the views and opinions. Homeopathic literature since long seems to be deficient in guidance about potency problem. Keeping this in mind the fundamentals of potency selection are taken for discussion in this book. The discussion has been kept limited to potencies in centesimal scale, as they are the most widely used potencies.

9. PLANNING AND PROGRAMMING OF TREATMENT

Potency selection and decision regarding repetition schedule form an integral part of planning and programming of treatment. Selection of a suitable remedy is just the first step in treating a patient. *Besides the remedy selection, the physician has to assess the probable acute remedies and intercurrent remedy that might be required in future during the treatment.* A thorough study of case record would reveal all these things to a rational homeopath. A physician has to judge in advance the type of response and the type of symptom changes to expect, after the first prescription is made. All this requires application of logic and philosophy.

■

CHAPTER 2

The Clinical Setup

- ❖ Financial Resources — 20
- ❖ Location/Site of Clinic — 22
- ❖ Interiors of the Clinic — 25
- ❖ Clinical Timings — 30
- ❖ Fee Structure — 32
- ❖ Physician's Attire — 33

CHAPTER 2

THE CLINICAL SETUP

Today there are hundreds of doctors coming out of various (allopathic, ayurvedic and homeopathic) medical colleges. Majority of them enter into private practice after their graduation. There are an average 10 clinics of various branches of medicine in any given market place. Most of the Indian cities seem to be saturated with nursing homes and clinics of varied branches of medicine. The number of practicing homeopaths has also increased by leaps and bounds in past few years. In such a situation only a few succeed in private practice. The rest are left blaming the stars. Apart from other reasons like lack of knowledge and skills etc., failures usually result from lack of attention and proper planning of the clinical setup.

The clinical setup and various factors related to it also play a small but important part in making up of a successful homeopath. Therefore planning and giving consideration to various aspects of a clinical setup is crucial to success in homeopathic practice. Most of the homeopaths find out through trial and error what is right and what is wrong with regards to their clinical setup. The budding homeopaths get guidance on all aspects except one, how to set up a homeopathic clinic? Many therefore fail inspite of having all that it takes to be a successful homeopath. A thorough consideration needs to be given to various aspects of a clinical setup when one decides to start a private clinic.

The six important aspects that need attention while starting a homeopathic clinic are:

1. Financial Resources.
2. Location / Site of Clinic.
3. Interiors of Clinic.
4. Clinical Timings.
5. Fee Structure.
6. Physician's Attire.

1. FINANCIAL RESOURCES

Finance is the backbone of any clinical setup. Nothing can be achieved without investing some amount of money in construction of a clinic as per professional requirements. An estimate needs to be prepared to find out the various costs involved in setting up a clinic. The estimate gives an idea of the total amount required for the clinical setup. It makes enormous sense to prepare a financial estimate in advance.

Following costs need to be taken into account while preparing a financial estimate for a clinical setup:

(i) **Furniture:** This includes doctor's chair, examination table, other tables and sitting arrangement for patients, cabinets, wooden cupboards for storage of medicines and case papers and filing cabinets etc.

(ii) **Medicines:** Homeopaths usually dispense medicines themselves hence cost of medicines needs to be taken into account. The cost of dilutions in various potencies, globules, sugar of milk, dispensing alcohol, plastic bottles and paper for preparing medicinal doses and crushing globules needs to be considered.

(iii) **Equipment:** Medical equipment like B.P. apparatus, weight machine, thermometer, torch, ear cannula, artery forceps, pair of scissors and dressing and bandage material etc.

(iv) **Stationary:** Letter pads, printed case record forms, follow-up sheets, visiting cards, files, writing material, rubber stamps and paper weight etc.

(v) **Electricity charges.**

(vi) **Telephone bill.**

(vii) **Assistant's and / or Receptionist's monthly salaries.**

(viii) **Professional tax.**

(ix) **Income tax.**

Besides giving an idea about the total amount required to start a clinic this estimate also helps to decide the fee structure. The fees per patient can be accessed by taking into consideration the above investment costs and recurring expenses for running a clinic. This may sound a bit too business like considering the fact that medicine is a profession and not a business but it is necessary to think over financial issues to avoid financial losses. Financial stability and management is must for survival of any profession which includes medical profession.

To take care of all these costs and recurring expenses a financial backup that is able to sustain a new homeopath for at least a year or two is must. This is because initially the income is going to be meagre and would not be sufficient to pay for all that is required for maintenance of a private clinic.

The time required to get settled and be financially stable is comparatively more in a homeopathic practice as compared to the allopathic one. Financial arrangements need to be made to take care of all these costs. The amount of money required to set up a private clinic can be arranged from various sources like:

(a) **One's own savings** (one can set aside certain amount from one's earnings through working in some hospital, clinic or medical facility after the internship period is over).

(b) **From family members / Parents**

(c) **Taking a loan from financial institutions** (like banks and finance companies).

2. LOCATION / SITE OF CLINIC

The proposed location of the clinic is one of the prime reasons/ factors which will have a direct impact on success or failure of the professional practice, as such it is all important to choose the site with due deliberation.

AN IDEAL LOCATION

A location or site can be ideal or otherwise for setting up a homeopathic clinic depending upon various factors. The factors which must be taken into account while deciding a suitable location are as follows:

- The clinic should be preferably situated at a place which is frequented by large number of people every day for various reasons. (A market place, main road, a busy street or a location near a bank or any other institution is ideal in this respect.)

- It is advantageous if the clinic is situated in such a place/area or locality where people know about homeopathy and are in the habit of taking homeopathic medicines for their day-to-day ailments.

- It should be located at a place, which is easily accessible to patients by various means of transport.

The Clinical Setup

- A homeopathic clinic (or any clinic for that matter) should be preferably on the ground floor or the building should have a lift, as the older people, severely disabled patients, and pregnant women may not be in a position to climb stairs.

- It does not matter if the clinic is located in an area or locality where there are already one or two famous and/or popular practicing homeopaths. But a new clinic should not be too near or next to such practitioner's establishment as in such a case there is always a danger of comparison in terms of experience, etc. and it may prove very damaging for a new practice.

The above criteria need to be kept in mind while deciding the site or location of a clinic. It is wise to make a survey of various localities in the city for at least few weeks, while searching a suitable location for a homeopathic clinic. After getting all the necessary information about the area or location one can make a logical and wise decision. It is better to take an alert and keen observing friend or a relative during the survey to take the details of the area that would prove helpful in making a decision. Given below is a list of various points that need to be kept in mind while doing a survey of a locality for setting up a homeopathic clinic.

- Number of practicing and popular homeopaths in the area.

- Number of other practicing physicians and specialists in the locality. *(This is important keeping in view the networking opportunities and team approach, in treating complicated cases, which might be needed in future).*

- The type of people residing in the area. *(Getting an idea about the socio-economic status, culture, customs and habits of the people in the area may prove useful in making a decision).*

- The transportation facilities available in the area. *(The distance of the nearest bus stand and railway station from the proposed site of a clinic. The proposed location should be convenient for outstation patients, otherwise they won't be willing and able to consult a physician due to inconvenience in transportation).*

- The distance of the location from the physician's place of residence. *(The place of practice should not be too far away from one's residence because sometimes the circumstances and conditions may require the physician's presence in his clinic urgently).* The traveling time and transportation costs need to be taken into account.
- Availability of other complementary medical facilities in the locality *(like pathology laboratory, radiologist, physiotherapy center, medical store and availability of homeopathic medicines, etc.).*
- Availability of advanced medical care. *(This is necessary, as sometimes in an emergency, a critical or serious patient needs to be referred to a nursing home or hospital immediately).*

Everyone does not have the luxury of owning or getting regular consulting room or clinic. Some homeopaths practice from their place of residence. It is good if a physician lives in a convenient location for his patients. A home practice has its own advantages. There is no extra rental or purchasing cost for the use of room or premises. One is more comfortable and relaxed at home. The cost of conveyance is saved. The timings can be flexible. However, there are some disadvantages also. A home practice does not give a very professional impression. Continuous pouring in of patients at inconvenient times might create a nuisance to the family. The drawing room, which is used as a consulting room in such cases will be required to be arranged daily which will be rather inconvenient for the members of the family. The kids playing and making noise may disturb the patients and toilet odours might be nauseous to the patients. In a home practice it is advisable to keep the home neat, clean, tidy and without any unpleasant odours.

3. INTERIORS OF THE CLINIC

A good clinic should have the basic facilities of toilet, drinking water and washbasin, etc. Cleanliness is expected of a doctor more than anyone else, therefore regular cleaning of toilet, basin and flooring is essential especially in a clinic.

The interiors of a clinic play a vital role in creating a good impression on patient's mind. The appearance and feel of the waiting room and consulting chamber should be neat, clean and comfortable. Cluttered condition of the room or clinic gives a look smaller than it really is. Patient forms opinions about the doctor and his practice from whatever he observes and feels during his visit to the clinic. The interiors and decor of the clinic reflect the personality of the practicing physician. It is therefore necessary to make sure that the clinic captures and reflects a physician's distinct personality throughout. This alone adds interest and individuality to the decor. A good interior decor can add to a clinic's feel and ambience.

Various factors need to be addressed while planning and designing the interiors of a clinic. They are:

(a) Lighting.
(b) Storage.
(c) Furniture.
(d) Equipments.
(e) Decor.

(a) LIGHTING

Components are:
- Sufficient lighting.
- Curtains.

Lighting should be used wisely. The consulting chamber should be such that there is sufficient daylight coming from the windows during day and good lamplight in evening hours. Poor lighting can give a very shabby look to the clinic's environment. Poor lighting can seriously hamper the look of the clinic and would also hamper the observation of the patient during case taking and physical examination.

Curtain fabric shades that allow control of the amount of light must be chosen. Soft translucent shades increase the amount of light and at the same time reduce the glare of computer screen if computer is in use. Dark curtain shades should be avoided as they severely hamper the incoming light and can make the room look badly illuminated. However dark curtains can be used in that part of clinic where physical examination is carried out and patient needs privacy.

Warmth can be quickly added to the clinical atmosphere with well-placed lighting options. It is said that lighting should be arranged to form a triangle. This can be used as a guide when placing or fixing lamps and tube lights. Lamp lighting provides more warmth and mood than overhead lighting. Spot lighting can be attractive when showing off an art. Lampshades that are slightly tan or yellow cast a warm glow to add mood and sophistication.

(b) STORAGE

Having adequate storage is the key to having an efficient workspace that is not cluttered. Adequate storage is required to store case records, files, stationary, medicines and other medical equipment. Storage equipments like filing cabinets etc. should be such that it occupies less space and looks more like furniture than stark office equipment. A secure filing system that can be locked is necessary for keeping case records in safe custody because patients want to be assured that their details remain confidential.

It is better to use a writing table with drawers, than using the one without them. Tables that have drawers store large amount of miscellaneous office items and thus help in avoiding a messy look.

The examination table can be converted into a good storage space by making concealed drawers and compartments below the top. Storing medicine bottles in a cabinet that does not conceal the bottles creates a more professional setting. The cupboard or cabinet that is used to store medicines should have a glass front so that patients can view the row of neatly arranged bottles. It is better to use amber coloured bottles for medicines rather than using white transparent bottles. Good storage space helps to keep the clinic more organised.

(c) FURNITURE

When buying furniture for a clinic it is important to make an educated choice because:

- The physician will probably live with it for a long time.
- Furniture can be one of the biggest investment one makes.
- Each piece should have a purpose, whether it is utilitarian or decorative.
- It is too expensive to replace large items of furniture therefore, furniture items should have the colours and style that will last through trends and time.

When buying furniture for a clinical setup, comfort is an important consideration. This is one area where one shouldn't be afraid to invest in. The cash one invests in quality items of office furniture will be repaid many times over with a high rate of productivity and efficiency. The physician's chair should be such that he can sit in a working posture for a longtime and the desk should be at a comfortable height. An overstuffed doctor's chair not only adds space but can add an inviting look to the consulting room.

The sitting arrangement for patient also needs to be equally comfortable. It is always better to have ample amount of chairs in the waiting room. In a busy clinic where lot of waiting is required to meet the doctor, patients may get irritated due to standing for long hours.

Smaller clinic can be made to look spacious by choosing small minimum furniture in order to avoid a cluttered look. The furniture one selects must be functional, not just pretty. It is best to make sure that each piece of furniture is positioned in a practical fashion.

(d) EQUIPMENTS

One should think carefully about what actually is necessary before buying any medical or other office equipment.

One should always check whether it fits into the space easily or not. It is better to buy the bare necessities and build on that, rather than buying a load of hi-tech equipment that one would hardly use. The most common mistake is buying a plethora of equipment only to find that one does not really need it or that it won't fit into the designated area. Buying second hand equipment should be considered to save some cash. Buying most essential medical equipments like B.P. apparatus, weight machine, stethoscope, etc. is must. A computer with good homeopathic software can help in reducing the time required for remedy selection in complicated cases. A computer can also help a physician in doing research on homeopathic topics and may aid in writing useful homeopathic literature. If one uses a computer, it is crucial that one keeps a backup of files on CDs. This will prevent loss of important data in case of computer failure. One may have all the case records stored in a computer but it is always a wise decision to have written records too. Too much dependence on computers can prove very disadvantageous to both physician and his patient if the machine fails suddenly.

(e) DECOR

Patients feel good and are impressed if the clinic is neatly decorated, well furnished and has an air of sophistication but, over decoration is unwanted as it may create an impression that the doctor's charges are too high and hence needs to be avoided. Moderate amount of decoration with bit of simplicity is all that is required.

A good effect is created by adding a personal touch so the physician should try to include some of his personality into the clinic's décor. It helps the patients to formulate an idea about the doctor's personality and interests. The best way to find out how to decorate your clinic is to think what would the patient expect to see in a clinic. Another way is to visit the clinics of other physicians to see and find out how they have decorated their clinics. A physician can make his clinic the best from beauty and artistic point of view without investing much money if he uses his creativity and imagination.

Decorating the interiors of a clinic is a matter of individual choices. There are no rules to follow. However there are certain general tips that can be useful while decorating.

Tips for decorating

- The decoration should be such that it gives a professional and sophisticated look.
- The decoration should reflect physician's personality.
- It is advisable to have a notice board in waiting room to display newspaper cuttings of news related to the physician and homeopathy. It is a good way of showing one's achievements. Photographs of physician receiving some award, degree or certificate, etc. can also be displayed. Such things help in creating the right impression on patient's mind.
- It is must to have a showcase displaying medical and homeopathic books in the consulting room. These books can be used for reference purpose when needed and also help in giving a qualified impression.

- It is better to put some flowers in flowerpot on physician's consulting table because flowers add a touch of freshness and an air of welcome.
- A rug or carpet laid on the floor helps to define an area and looks attractive and warm.
- It is better to use pastel colours as they are most effective in creating a peaceful setting and increase the lightness of the rooms. Dark colours make the rooms look smaller than they really are therefore dark colours should be avoided. White and cream are best for a clinical setup. Shades of gray can also add to the clinical look. For the fullest effect of space one should not paint the walls the same colour as the ceiling. Pastel colour can be used for walls and the ceiling can be covered with clean white finish. White ceiling helps to reflect much needed light. The lighter the room, the bigger it appears.
- Artwork and photographs should be hung at eye level. At an eye level, the pieces can be appreciated and can be a part of room's décor.
- The pleasant smell of scented candles or incense sticks helps to add freshness and cool atmosphere.
- Large or medium sized mirrors when fixed at a suitable place give an illusion of a larger space than it actually is. Mirrors can be used where the space is small and one wants to make it look bigger.
- House plants and trailing vines in a basket placed at suitable place (especially at corners) can help in bringing nature to one's workspace.

4. CLINICAL TIMINGS

The clinical timings have to be decided keeping in mind patient's convenience. If this is not done physician looses many potential patients. It is observed that afternoon hours are most

The Clinical Setup   31

unsuitable as most of the people are busy with their daily duties. Usually the clinical timings for majority of the clinics are in morning and evening. Evening timings are more popular as most of the people especially office goers have free time in evening. Timings such as morning 9 to 12 and evening 6 to 9 are suitable and common with majority of general practitioners. However, some variations in these routine timings need to be made according to the type of people in the locality, their habits and needs.

Keeping the clinic open on Sundays is a good idea as almost everybody has time on Sunday. But if one keeps his clinic open on Sunday he should think of some alternative weekday as a holiday. One day rest in a week is must for every physician. Keeping clinic open on all 7 days of the week can prove very strenuous and taxing to a physician mentally as well as physically and hence is not advisable.

In the beginning years of practice a homeopath may be required to see a patient at most odd and unsuitable time of the day, but as the practice progresses he will have better command over the hours when he can make himself available to his patients. A new homeopath should always welcome an appointment even if it is at a most inconvenient time. He should never try to escape a home visit, when a bedridden patient needs urgent help even if it is in odd hours of night. It is not advisable to keep mobile off in night hours fearing that patients may bother at night. If someone calls a doctor in odd night hours, it means he really needs help. A good homeopath should always encourage his patients to call whenever they need help, because not hearing from patients at all is worse than getting complaints. A good physician is the one who is easily accessible to his patients even when he is not in the clinic.

A homeopath should never be in a hurry to go home in the closing hours of clinic, as there is always a possibility of getting a new patient if one stays a bit longer in clinic. A homeopath should be very disciplined and particular about timings. Getting late to the clinic should be avoided as one may loose an important patient every time one gets late.

5. FEE STRUCTURE

The question of fees is a complex one to answer. The doctor's charges in all parts of the world especially in a country like India are continuously on the rise. People want and need an affordable treatment. Homeopathy is a good option in this situation.

A genuine homeopath has to work harder to give results, as homeopathy is 'individual' medicine. There are no specifics. Each case is a new case. A detailed case taking and remedial diagnosis requires hard work. Apart from this, investment costs are involved in setting up a private clinic, which need consideration while deciding the fees. A present day homeopath cannot afford to charge too less like his predecessors did. If he charges high, again there is a problem. If the fee is exorbitant then there is likelihood of a physician going beyond patient's range of affordability. Thus, he may loose patients due to high fees.

If one keeps his fees too low patients may think that there is a lack of both quality and experience or they may conclude that the physician is desperate for their business. The charges should never be too low, because if a physician himself does not value his services, patients also won't value his services.

Best way is to be moderate in charging a fees. One should charge what one is worth. To settle the question of fees, one must first find out what the other homeopaths in the area are charging. One may find differences in the fee structure of various homeopaths in a given locality. The motive behind finding what others charge is to get the idea about the range of fees that are appropriate to the location of practice and the pathy. It is advisable to keep the fees with in this range obtained from market research.

In case the people in the area of practice are in the habit of calling a doctor home for every trivial complaint, the home visit fees should be better on a higher side. This is done to curtail patients who make unnecessary demand of home visit. However, when the patient is seriously ill and not in a position to visit the clinic he should not be charged very high for a home visit. The home visit fees should be inclusive of the additional amount for traveling in terms of time and costs. One should not avoid home visits, as they can be a source of additional monetary gains if no one else is offering such a service.

6. PHYSICIAN'S ATTIRE

Attire or clothing plays an important role in building a person's personality. It is common to find people judging others from the type of attire worn. There are many things that go to make a complete doctor, what he wears is one of them. There is a saying that, "Clothing makes a man." It is equally true for a doctor as it is for any person. Physician's attire is one of the factors, which contributes in creating a good impression in patient's mind. An attire or dress indicates a physician's social status and personality.

Neat and clean attire helps the physician to feel confident. A doctor's dress need not be very stylish or fashionable. It should be neat, clean and comfortable. The costume worn should gives a professional look. Wearing a tie can add to the professional look. If one wears shoes then they should always be polished.

A patient who is referred by another patient has already formed an image about the doctor from the description given by the referring patient. When he actually arrives at the clinic he expects the doctor's image and personality to comply with his preconceived notions about the doctor. If the case is not so he may get a bit disappointed. This can have a negative effect on that particular patient's belief and confidence about the doctor and his treatment. ■

CHAPTER 3

Homeopathic Physician - Redefined

CHAPTER 3

HOMEOPATHIC PHYSICIAN - REDEFINED

The most important constituent of homeopathic practice is the homeopathic physician himself. It is he who is responsible for curing diseases by the application of the law of similars and therefore it is he who brings glory to his science and establishes faith in it. It, therefore, naturally follows that it is the homeopathician himself who is responsible for boosting the image of the science he practices. If he succeeds the science succeeds, but if he fails, his failure is seen as the failure of the science. But the science of homeopathy which is based on certain principles cannot be blamed for the failure; it is the physician who fails not the science. Thus, a lot of what is termed as homeopathic practice depends upon this pivotal figure, the homeopathic physician.

Homeopathy since the time of Hahnemann has seen many a medical men and homeopathic graduates prescribing 'white pills' and calling themselves 'homeopaths', but very few of them can be truly called as 'homeopathic physicians'. There has only been a quantitative and not qualitative rise in the homeopathic practitioners. Consequently, quality of homeopathic physicians has seriously deteriorated, while the number of charlatans has increased. A re-investigation of the term 'homeopathic physician' will make it obvious that there is dearth of men of substance and the number of genuine homeopathic physicians is perpetually dwindling. Only a microscopic number of physicians practice Hahnemannian homeopathy. We have forgotten what is meant by the term 'True Practitioner of the Healing Art.' This makes it compulsory to find out who is a genuine homeopathic physician. What is he expected to know ? What is he expected to do ? What makes him successful ? Why he fails in his duty? To answer all these questions we would have to review, reinvestigate & redefine the term 'Homeopathic Physician'.

Dr. Hahnemann in the 3rd aphorism of Organon of Medicine expects the true practitioner to have a command over the science of nosological diagnosis, that is medicine, and a clear idea about the portraits of various drugs enlisted in homeopathic materia medica. Hahnemann does not forgets that the physician must know the application of homeopathic laws and application of medicines according to law of similars for curing the sick. He adds that for successful application of the law of similars it is a must that the physician should be an unprejudiced observer.

Kent in his lesser writings defines the homeopathic physician as the "one who adds to his knowledge of medicine a special knowledge of homeopathic therapeutics and observes the law of similars". He further adds that, "the homeopathic physician is one who prescribes single remedy in minimum dose in potentized form, selected according to law of similars". His message is " Men have become great in homeopathy in following the principles laid down in Hahnemann's Organon, in teaching, translating, compiling and prescribing, but not a single man has become great by using tinctures, compound tablets, or ignoring the doctrines of potentization." Kent distinguishes a physician who seems to be a homeopath from the one who is a genuine homeopath. To put it in his own words, *" I would prefer an allopath to one who professes* to be a homeopath but does not know enough homeopathy to practice it. *If the doctor has not the grit to withstand the cries of the family, the criticism of friends, the threatening of his pocketbook & of his bread and butter he will not practice homeopathy very long. An honest man does not fear these things ".* What Kent meant was that a genuine physician strictly follows and applies all the cardinal principles of homeopathy and for doing so possesses the required knowledge in an adequate amount.

While Stuart Close has quite practically stated that a homeopathic physician is the representative of the 'pathy', and therefore the success of the 'pathy' depends upon the success of its representative, the physician. It is therefore necessary that the physician gains technical proficiency in the application of principles and laws that govern the science of homeopathy. According to him a true homeopath must have the qualities of courage, honesty, fidelity to a high ideal and a right point of view. By right point of view he means the homeopathic point of view, where the individual suffering from the disease is of utmost importance than the disease itself, or the part affected by the disease. Dr. Close makes it clear that, "A mere formal knowledge of the law of cure and the technique of prescribing does not make a homeopathic physician in the true sense of the word." He wants that the spirit of homeopathy should be incarnated in every follower and feels that every beginner in homeopathy should have the desire to make the laws and teachings of homeopathy the ruling influence of his life.

Roberts also stresses the same points which Hahnemann and Kent stressed on but in addition remarks that homeopathic physician is the one who follows the laws regardless of pressure or influence, because it is the principles which he follows stabilize him and make him sure in his work. From this we can conclude that following the laws and principles of homeopathy definitely plays a major role in the degree of confidence in homeopathic prescribing.

Therefore only men with determination and philosophical bent of mind can practice 'Hahnemannian homeopathy' in truest sense of the term. According to Roberts, a true homeopath is the one who does not ask what homeopathy can do for him but tries to do what he can for the science of homeopathy.

According to Dr. M.L. Dhawale, "A homeopathic physician is one who perceives the man behind the illness and that too in an unprejudiced manner, to find the exact correspondence of the portrait of disease with one amongst the many, stored by him in his memory store constantly replenished through active clinical experience." He states that homeopathy can't survive in the absence of efficient results. He is absolutely right when he says homeopathy is philosophy in action. The men we call stalwarts in homeopathy have clearly underlined what the term homeopathic physician means.

All of them have emphasized that a homeopathic physician should be an efficient one, one who is competent enough to give results strictly following the principles laid down by Hahnemann, only then he can be called as the true practitioner or a genuine homeopath. Everyone agrees that 'results' are must for survival of homeopathy and homeopath, but the definition of 'results' varies with every individual physician. What does a homeopath understands by the term 'results' needs to be investigated. For some results means relieving the patient of his complaints, for others it is recovery of the patient, while for very few physicians the term results means curing the patient of his disease. So, the physicians who want to give their patients 'relief' (only relief no cure) settle for specifics and shortcuts and other products designed for 'relief.' They blame the single remedies for being unable to give 'quick relief to the patient.' But homeopathy cannot be blamed for the inefficiency of the one who practices it. As the 'bad workman quarrels with his tools' similarly shifting the blame on the 'pathy' is an escape route, taken by these physicians, true homeopath is the one who knows how to use his therapeutic armamentarium and never blame the instruments for his failures.

In every homeopath lies the potential to develop himself as an efficient physician but only the one who works hard for it and takes a proper route to success can be termed as a genuine homeopathic physician. Only such an efficient physician can "perceive the man behind the illness" as enunciated by Dr. Dhawale. Hahnemann had once aptly remarked that, "We have to do with an art whose end is saving of human life, any neglect to make ourselves thoroughly masters of it becomes a crime." A true homeopathic physician is the master of the system of medicine he practices. Thus performance oriented learning is the first step in making of a genuine homeopath. It is precisely this, which is seriously lacking in the homeopathic medical education and it has proved to be a major stumbling block to the process of making an efficient homeopath. It is therefore the lack of it which is the cause of production of large majority of 'pseudo-homeopaths' for whom the crutches of homeopathic patents, combinations, and pathological prescribing, become inevitable.

- Strict follower of Hahnemannian principles.
- Performance oriented learning.
- Persistent hard work.

Hahnemann has criticized such physicians who appear to be homeopaths in footnote to aphorism No. 67. These are the physicians who do not hesitate to compromise with the principles, which are the foundation of the pathy of similars. We should try to be masters of what we practice.

It is our duty and the duty of teachers is to teach us 'applied homeopathy'; only then can we do justice to the patients, who come to us to be relieved of their suffering. It is only when we are efficient then and then would our patients have full faith in us and our pathy. Thus efficiency is like oxygen to homeopathy and the homeopath, necessary for the survival of both.

Homeopathy demands total commitment, hence persistent efforts are must if the physician wants to perfect the art of efficient prescribing. Homeopathic physicians can never afford to be complacent. Hard work is needed for giving good results repeatedly. Homeopathy is not for the indolent and lazy men. Even Hahnemann has warned homeopaths from being indolent. Hahnemann in preface to first edition of Organon of Medicine says that, *"I must warn the reader that indolence, love of ease and obstinacy preclude effective service at the alter of truth, and only freedom from prejudice and untiring zeal qualify for the most sacred of all human occupations, the practice of true system of medicine."* Thus we see here how he has described here the eligibility and qualifications necessary for being a genuine homeopathic physician. It thus becomes obvious that a homeopath is a student for lifetime; he should always add to his knowledge of medicine, allied sciences and homeopathy, and at no point of time should he get satisfied with his efforts at practicing Hahnemannian homeopathy. Motivation coupled with devotion and commitment to the science and a desire for excellence are essential prerequisites for the one who wishes to be a genuine homeopath.

From this elaborate investigation, we can summarize the prerequisites that play a major role in making of a 'True Homeopathic Physician.' A student who aspires to be a genuine physician of the Hahnemannian art of healing should try to concentrate on the five 'P's which are very essential.

1. Performance oriented learning.
2. Persistent efforts.
3. Philosophical bent of mind.
4. Practical approach to homeopathic philosophy.
5. Patience to an immense degree.

The first 'P' performance oriented learning is difficult find and hence rarely witnessed. Unfortunately homeopathic education especially in India where homeopathy is recognized by Government leaves much to be desired in this respect. A performance-oriented learning is that type of learning, which makes a student able to perform well in a practical situation. It enables the student to handle various types of cases with ease and confidence. It does not depend totally upon the learner. The educational institution has an equal responsibility too. A sound infrastructure capable of providing a student all the facilities, study material including O.P.D. and I.P.D. patients is a must. Most of homeopathic institutions lack in basic infrastructure and the number of patients necessary for clinical training of a homeopath are also grossly lacking. Besides this, bedside teaching also requires skilled lecturers, which may not be available in some of these institutions. In case a student gets attached to any private homeopathic clinic and if his 'Guru' is competent and a genuine homeopath then he too learns good homeopathy and if his teacher himself is not an efficient performer the student cannot develop as a competent homeopath from 'learning' at such a private clinic. This makes performance-oriented learning highly individualistic. Hence the clinical training gained by every homeopathic student varies with the physician who guides him in a private clinic. All this again contributes to the growing number of 'pseudo-homeopaths. The one who wishes to be a competent practitioner should make his choices thoughtfully if he wishes to learn quality homeopathy. Making careful choices and getting associated with scientific practitioners is not enough. Learning involves assimilating from a number of sources. If one is truly interested in knowing how to practice homeopathy scientifically then there is voluminous information around him. One needs to pick it up. A child like curiosity is necessary unless one fills up his bag with therapeutic armamentarium one would not be able to use it to cure patients when necessary.

Another way out is the clinical training centers that are doing commendable job in imparting practical knowledge to a student physician. In this respect clinical training center established by Dr. George Vithoulkas and the other by Dr. Alfons Geukens in Belgium deserve special appreciation. In India I.C.R. (Institute of Clinical Research) is also imparting clinical training. *(For contact details and addresses of these clinical training centers see the last chapter of this book).* Such organizations are contributing a lot in giving homeopathy competent and law-abiding homeopaths. Such clinical training is a must, as only this kind of learning will bridge the gap between theory and practice. In such kind of training a student physician sees good results and well taken cases in practice which can prove very motivating for performance-oriented learning. Such centers are the places where it is easy to study the homeopathic follow up of long term cases. A training of 3 to 5 years in such center would definitely make the budding homeopath capable of handling most of the cases in practice with success.

Knowledge of the disease being an essential prerequisite for perceiving the patient, it becomes necessary for a neophyte to master the art of diagnosing diseases. The best way to do this is spending some time under the guidance of proficient specialists of various types for example, skin specialists, E.N.T. surgeons, psychiatrist, a pediatrician, etc. before the homeopathic clinical training. One need not forget that learning is a continuous process for a homeopathic physician. Even a busy and experienced homeopath cannot afford to totally cut himself from books and learning. To achieve perfection an unending thirst for knowledge is a must for a true homeopath. Boenninghausen, well aware of the complexities and vastness of science of homeopathy, advises busy physicians in his article 'Old and New Matters' to avoid being complacent. He states that memory needs repeated freshening up and therefore a homeopath should regularly refer books, especially various repertories and materia medica. To put it in his words,

"But outside of these regular hours of recreation now and then, according as his time is more or less occupied by those seeking his aid, he now and then will find some moments of leisure which his profession makes it his duty to employ in enlarging and perfecting his knowledge of his self selected calling."

The last 'P' patience is also a must for a genuine homeopath. On the road to success and perfection one may come across initial disappointments and failures especially in a highly demanding science like homeopathy. However, persistent efforts are a must if one wishes to develop the potential for genuine and successful homeopathic practice. Along with persistent efforts an effective synchronization of learning, understanding and implementing what is learned and understood is also necessary. All knowledge is useless without application.

Patience, persistent efforts and philosophical bent of mind are the preliminary requisitions for successful implementation of homeopathic philosophy in practice. Practical approach to homeopathic philosophy incorporates proper and logical interpretation of the homeopathic doctrine. Balanced interpretation of homeopathic principles requires what Hahnemann calls an 'unprejudiced observation' and sound logic. An illogical interpretation of homeopathic principles and philosophy would surely confuse a budding homeopath.

Therefore, introspection into whether what is being interpreted from the books of philosophy is rightly interpreted or not is required. Hence a budding homeopath should guard himself against these 'P's:

1. Prejudiced observation,
2. Pseudo-homeopathic approach and
3. Pseudo-homeopathic prescribing.

Homeopathic practice is a serious business. It demands a physician tobe aware of his responsibilities because a life is at

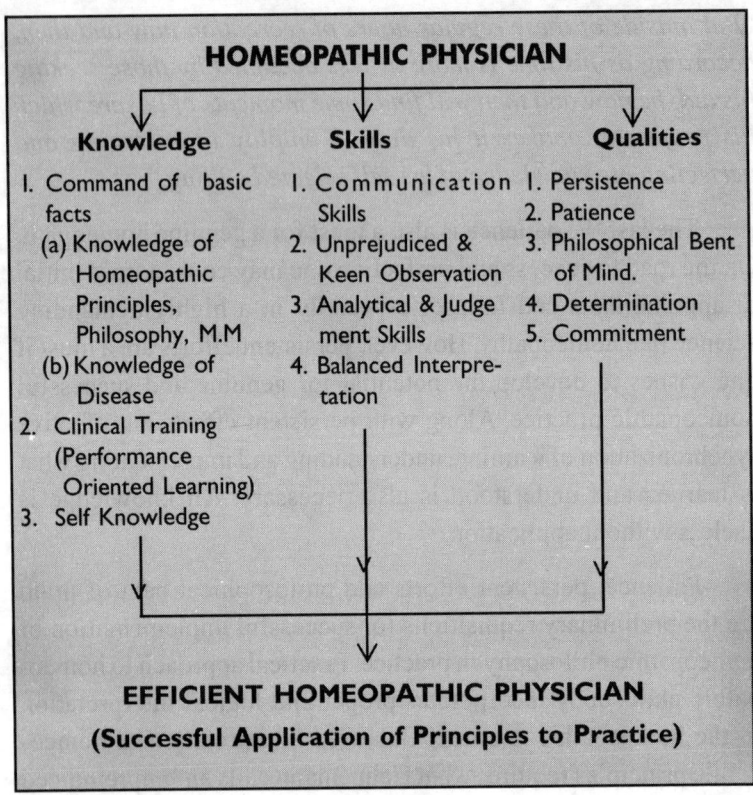

stake. It demands a physician who refuses to entertain casual attitude towards practice and tries to gain mastery over his science. Unfortunately a very dismal number of physicians are aware of these things. Homeopathy needs strong men, men of substance, of principles and character and honest men as its practitioners. Homeopathy gives more than enough to a dedicated homeopath. But practicing homeopathy with principles is like swimming against the current. It involves considerable hard work for which very few of the present day student-homeopaths may be ready. All the laws and principles that we as a student learn from the 'Bible of Homeopathy' (The Organon) are for application in practice. We should know that theory and practice are same; it is we who divide them in separate compartments.

Homeopathic physician - Redefined

It won't be out of place to quote a few lines from Jeremy Sherr's article 'Medicine of the Future', which beautifully explains which type of physician deserves the title of 'Homeopath.' He writes, *"There are homeopaths, and then there are those who use potentized remedies. There are homeopaths, and then there are those who prescribe hundreds of remedies per patient on passing whims. There are homeopaths, and then there are those who prescribe for single organs, fail to take the case, deny provings, combine remedies. There are homeopaths and then there are those who hold Nux vomica in one hand and steroids in the other. There are homeopaths, and then there are those who use only a small and convenient portion of the principles, which define our science. It is these dabblers who should define themselves with another name. The title of homeopath needs no adjective and belongs to those who practice the totality of its principles."*

Homeopathy demands a physician who firmly believes in its principles and has got the capacity to incorporate them in his practice, in spite of whatever cost he may have to pay for doing so. It is then, that he will have the right to call himself 'True Therapist of the Art of Similars' that is the "Homeopathic Physician."

■

CHAPTER 4

Secrets of Effective Case-Taking

- ❖ Introduction — 51
- ❖ Difficulties in Conducting Inquiry — 53
- ❖ Before the Clinical Session — 58
- ❖ Art of Communication — 60
- ❖ Establishing 'Rapport' and Skilled Listening — 61
- ❖ Five Key Aspects of Clinical Interview — 66
- ❖ Inquiry in Pediatric Cases — 74
- ❖ Physical Examination — 78
- ❖ Documentation in Homeopathic Practice — 80

CHAPTER 4

SECRETS OF EFFECTIVE CASE-TAKING

INTRODUCTION

The first step in treating the patient is case-taking or recording information, which constitutes the most important part of homeopathic practice. Unfortunately it still remains the most neglected part in both the homeopathic training as well as clinical application. A homeopath cannot do his best in treating a patient without thorough case taking. He is totally handicapped if there is paucity of information. Thus it becomes very important to be well conversant with all the aspects of case taking. Let us investigate—What is case taking? Why people fail in it? and What are the secrets of effective case taking?

Case taking can be defined as a science and art of collecting and recording information from the patient and his associates in order to arrive at a logical conclusion regarding to the nosological diagnosis, prognosis and the choice of remedy. The homeopathic fraternity in general is well conversant with the theoretical aspect of case taking but the practical implications of the concept of case taking are yet a mystery for many. Every true homeopath wants to know 'what lies beneath' an effective clinical interview. Many budding as well as practicing homeopaths consider case taking as a laborious, time-consuming, impractical and most difficult task. The prejudices against case taking are abundant. Good case taking is not as enigmatic as it seems and neither impossible, the more you get exposed to it and indulge in it the more easier it gets for you.

Key to effective case taking lies in application of the views of various stalwarts in practice. But application of theory in practice is the most difficult part, particularly when it comes to thorough case taking, that is why clinical investigation in homeopathic practice is called an art by one and all. This art like any other art needs a skilled individual to perform it, but unfortunately the level of skill varies with every individual homeopath and exactly here lies the crux of the problem. Everyone agrees that it is the most important part of homeopathic practice and first step towards selection of right remedy and curing the patient. But skilled interrogation is least understood and lesser applied by the majority of homeopaths. The art of case taking can be mastered only after getting exposed to several clinical interviews under the guidance of an experienced senior homeopath. But such opportunities are very few as the patient does not want any other person except the physician in the consulting room, and he has a right to expect that. Thus in most of the cases this art like any other art has to be developed by the concerned physician himself, although books and teachers can make the physician's job a bit easier.

I would rather call it a science that needs an artist. In case taking, the information is collected on certain predetermined parameters, i.e. a predetermined standardized format hence it can be called as a science, but only a skilled physician can get what he wants out of this procedure hence it is an art. Collecting evidence to pinpoint the remedy is the most important part of the homeopathic practice and therefore any negligence, prejudice or lack of skill on the part of physician would result in failures and complications in the case. The key to successful homeopathic practice lies in giving sufficient time for conducting inquiry.

Hahnemann himself devoted at least 30 to 45 minutes for case taking. Jotting down few lines on a piece of paper and calling it case taking is worthless. With such a habit the physician can only 'give results' but would never be in a position to cure his cases according to Hering's law of cure.

DIFFICULTIES IN CONDUCTING INQUIRY

Receiving the case is the most important as well as most difficult part of homeopathic practice. Even for an experienced and skilled homeopath there lie many obstacles in getting the required information, while for a beginner difficulties abound in both acute as well as chronic cases. These difficulties can be broadly divided into the obstacles due to patient and those due to physician.

1. OBSTACLES DUE TO PATIENT

- Patient accustomed to allopathic mode of treatment.
- Patient irritated by enquiries.
- Absence of face to face confrontation with the patient.
- Secretive patients.
- Exaggerating patients.
- Bashful patients.
- Indolent patients.
- Circumstantial problems.
- Patient unaware of homeopathic questionnaire and its importance.

Basic difficulty lies in the fact that majority of population is accustomed to allopathic mode of concentrating on physical examination and prescribing on its basis. An allopath never expects a detailed narration of complaints and if a patient tries to elaborate he is quickly discouraged which makes him think that only physical examination and few broad expressions for telling his problems are sufficient for a physician for prescription making. While some patients, 'the educated' amongst them bring earlier prescriptions, X-rays, reports of laboratory tests and are under the impression that they are providing great help to their homeopath by doing so. Precisely this attitude of the patient is a major block in case taking.

Some patients who have never observed many things about themselves get irritated when the physician inquires about the details such as quantity of sweat, stains and odour of sweat, and the quantity of water consumed or thirst, etc. These questions seem ridiculous to them, as they are not accustomed to homeopathic method of inquiry.

Since the time of Hahnemann, this has been the difficulty posed by those who are seeking homeopathic treatment for the first time. Even a homeopathic stalwart like, Dr. J.T. Kent found the questions of a homeopath Dr. Phelan as odd, seemingly inappropriate and ridiculous. It was Dr. Kent's first encounter with the homeopathic way of taking a case. It is after his wife was successfully cured, he realised how important the questions were.

In an acute case if the complaints are severe and violent many a times the patient is not brought to the clinic and the matter is reported by his relatives who use only general terms like high fever, headache, bodyache, etc. to describe the patients condition. Such a description serves no purpose for a homeopath. Even if he tries to inquire about other details, the relatives are not in a position to answer his queries. If the patient lives far off the physician cannot visit him to take stock of the situation. Sometimes even repeated requests to bring patient to the clinic fall on deaf ears. When the physician visits such a patient, due to the severity of complaints patient is not in a mental condition to answer his queries properly, and this usually results in his best efforts failing to give him the necessary information.

Then there are those patients who are secretive and never reveal their emotional side to the physician. Instead these 'hard nuts to crack' patients advice the physician to concentrate on 'complaints' rather than venturing into their private life, because for them it is the body which is ill and needs treatment, while mind is a separate compartment.

The patients, who have a tendency to exaggerate their complaints and describe them in vivid colours, hinder the process of getting the facts about the case. They do so under impression that such description would make the physician pay more attention to their case. They also feel that such vivid description would get them 'high power medicine' as they call it, so as to get quickly relieved of their complaints.

The bashful patients hide complaints belonging to sexual sphere and those complaints that they feel will land them in an awkward situation while the others forget certain symptoms as they are used to them. Similarly indolent patients also use vague terms and forget the details. Hahnemann has described these varieties of patients in paragraphs no. 96 to 98 of Organon of Medicine.

With the changing times certain miscellaneous hindrances, which I would call circumstantial problems seem to play a role in obstructing facts. For example, a lady using sanitary pads would not be in a position to tell whether the menstrual stains are washable or not. Similarly a man belonging to nuclear family is in most of the cases totally unaware of the sufferings and illnesses of his kith and kin. This prevents the family history from being known to the concerned physician.

The difficulty posed by those patients who are not accustomed to homeopathic mode of inquiry or those who are approaching a homeopath for the first time can be reduced by making them acquainted with the requirements of homeopathic practice for treating a chronic case. Such patients should be made aware of the importance of detailed case taking and its role in their treatment. The type of information required can be indicated by way of a history form.

The history form should be given to the patient prior to his appointment, so that he can go through it and furnish the required information in writing to the treating physician.

Patient should be encouraged to write a free account of his troubles as they occur to him at the time of writing. The patient should be advised to append to his history, copies of previous reports and treatments and the original report on the present medical state furnished by his earlier physician.

After receiving the history form from the patient the physician should go through it and make a note of any incomplete information which will have to be completed by careful subsequent enquiry. Areas, which have been avoided, should be noted. The physician must decide whether he should pursue this point immediately or wait for a more opportune time.

2. OBSTACLES DUE TO PHYSICIAN HIMSELF

- Laziness.
- Neophyte.
- Diagnostic and 'specific' prescribers.
- Lame excuses by physician.
- Shy attitude.
- Lack of training.

Secrets of Effective Case-taking

The lazy physicians who are always in search of easy ways to practice homeopathy are averse to detailed case taking. These physicians rush up the whole process in just 10-15 minutes and claim that they do a detailed case taking of every patient that visits them. They are the ones who put questions on remedy lines and this they think would lead them quickly to the simillimum. This is what can be termed as prejudiced inquiry.

The beginners are poor investigators partly due to lack of guidance as regards to 'How to do it'? Hence their case record is grossly deficient.

The diagnostic prescribers and the believers in 'homeopathic specifics' believe that case taking has only educational value and it is not for practical application. While some physicians give excuses for not following the interrogation procedure by saying that, "The patient of today has no time for such a prolonged interview session." Then there are those who carry out the case taking process with all its details but due to modesty and shyness avoid inquiry into the sexual sphere and personal matters of the patient. Similarly there are other physicians who also conduct a detailed inquiry but lack of tact, training and tenacity make them incapable of getting the emotional side of the case or mental symptoms and this makes case taking a tedious business for them.

This elaborated description of difficulties in interrogation should not make the reader think that these obstacles cannot be overcome. This does not mean that the physician should use these difficulties as excuses to hide his lack of skill and lack of experience in handling the interview process. It is in the ability to get over these impediments, lies the art of case taking which every true homeopath should try to develop, although it is a difficult job that may take few years. Books and masters are always there to guide him in his efforts to become a master investigator.

BEFORE THE CLINICAL SESSION

Essential components are:
- Case-taking proforma.
- Interview chamber.
- Impression by patient.
- Reputation of physician.
- Patient's expectation.

The case taking should be done usually at the beginning of clinical hours as the physician is fresh and the possibility of disturbances in the form of patients is less. Case taking carried out in the ending hours of clinical time when the practitioner is about to leave for home always proves fruitless in terms of information obtained. This happens because the physician is in a hurry to go home so he rushes up the whole process, thus making the case taking a formality. Case taking should preferably be done after giving a prior appointment to the patient. In the first visit the patients are usually not fully aware of the type of detailed information required for homeopathic treatment. Patients may be given a case taking form in their first visit. The form includes all the information required by the homeopath and therefore, gives patients a fair idea of the type of inquiry going to be carried out on the appointment day. The physician should be ready with blank format of case taking 10 to 15 minutes prior to the appointment time on the appointment day.

According to Dr. George Vithoulkas the place where the interview is going to be carried out is also equally important. Usually the physician's chamber is the place where the clinical interview is carried out. The environment should be quiet and such that the interruptions are minimum. The doctor's chamber should be preferably sound proof, so as to give the patient a feel of complete privacy; this can be done by closing the door or putting on the curtains without hampering the light coming in, before the interview begins. Noise interruption and changes in illumination are commonest distracters which should be minimum. A physician who is frequently interrupted by his assistant and other patients would not be able to concentrate on the interview. Frequent interruptions break the link of thoughts in patients mind while narrating his complaints; it is sure to spoil case recording. Case taking, therefore, should be preferably scheduled at the time when other regular patients are minimal. Sometimes this may not be possible, as the patients own daily schedule may not allow him to be present for the case taking when the physician desires. This problem can be handled by mutual understanding between the physician and the patient.

Office décor, furnishings, layout, lighting, and ventilation etc. should be designed with the patient's comfort as the primary consideration along with functional needs of the physician. All the efforts to minimize the waiting period are must although it is a difficult task in a busy clinic as prolonged waiting often irritates the patient, and such an irritated patient would naturally be less cooperative while case taking. Patient can be made comfortable in waiting room by providing reading material such as magazines and newspapers. Basic facilities like drinking water and toilet should be made available.

The proverb first impression is the last impression proves to be true even in homeopathic consultation. Actually the first impression is the 'lasting impression.'

The first impressions play a major role in opinion formation. Within the first few moments after his entry into physician's office, the patient starts forming his impressions about the physician. He forms it from what he sees in the consulting room i.e. the physician's appearance, his facial expression, arrangement of things, etc. These are the things that are available to him. A good impression in the first visit itself greatly helps in building patient's confidence. Physician's look therefore should inspire confidence;

he should appear to be trustworthy, efficient and should try to be himself. Sincerity of heart and positive attitude are enough for this purpose.

When a known patient visits for follow up he should be greeted with a smile. The patient feels acknowledged when he receives a smile from the physician. A smile conveys I know you, I remember your case, and I am interested in you as a patient. Patient wants a sympathetic, friendly, concerned and interested physician. One should never forget that, *"a patient does not care how much the physician knows, until he knows how much the physician cares."*

There is another saying, which a homeopath must remember that is, "when the patient enters my office I go out." What it means is that whatever the patient sees, hears, or observes while he is in physicians chamber, may it be good or bad is going to be carried out with him and naturally that is what the community is going to know about the physician. If it is good it will prove helpful in establishing, what is called, 'The reputation of the physician.'

Patient expects:
- A friendly, compassionate, sympathetic & interested physician.
- A physician who can feel his sufferings as he himself is feeling.
- A physician who views him as a 'suffering human being and not as a body with some faults in its organs.'

ART OF COMMUNICATION

Voltaire once remarked, "Doctors pour drugs of which they know little, to cure diseases of which they know less, into human beings of whom they know nothing." Whether what he said referred to only allopaths or all types of physicians including homeopaths we do not know. But we surely know that 'knowing the human beings' is most important business of a homeopath. Homeopathic interrogation is all about *'knowing the man (individual) behind the illness.'* However, it is easier said than done. It is difficult to achieve and cannot be achieved without tactful communication. Communicating with the patient is a sensitive and skilful procedure. Physician's attitude and approach to case taking is the deciding factor in the amount and quality of information that is going to be collected and recorded during the clinical interview. Everything depends on how he views the procedure of case taking. A physician who finds it a laborious, time consuming and impractical task would reduce the case taking to a mere formality carried out to pose as a scientific homeopath.

But the physician who views it as a social intercourse and approaches the patient as if he is meeting a friend who needs help proves successful in gathering all the vital evidences in the case. It is this approach, practiced over a period of years is what makes him a master observer and a master investigator.

ESTABLISHING 'RAPPORT' AND SKILLED LISTENING

Important constituents are:

- Case-taking.
- Patient listening.
- Concentration.
- Attentiveness.
- Avoid interruption.
- Positive body language.
- Physician's manners.
- Physician's expressions.
- Regular eye-contact.
- Avoid prejudiced observation.

- Avoid leading questions.
- Avoid suggestive questions.
- Observe patient's facial expressions.
- Vivid description of complaints within limited time.
- Mental symptoms.

Effective communication that is central to the concept of case taking will have to be cultivated by the physician himself. However there are certain general guidelines that can prove helpful in this regard. The most important tip regarding effective communication is that the case taking should not be a question-answer session. Homeopathic case-taking is not an interview for a job appointment, it is a social intercourse this should never be forgotten. It is better to carry out the case taking in the form of conversation or discussion. The inquiry should not be merely mechanical and formal as the lawyers do in court. Establishing 'the rapport' should be the prime aim in the beginning of the interview. The word rapport means 'in close relationship' or in sympathy. Rapport is the 'tuning in' of the physician with the frequency of the patient. Physician has to adjust himself according to the needs, demands and the type of individual he is investigating. Physician's approach will vary with the case in consideration. Rapport is like grease, it lubricates doctor-patient relationship.

Dr. Bernard S. Siegel, a Connecticut surgeon in his article on doctor-patient relationship states, " I want to see doctors put their desks against the wall and step into life and the world of the patient, and stop being a tourist and become a native in a new land." For a homeopath stepping into 'patients world' is a must to get the emotional side of the case. A patient will allow a doctor to enter in to his emotional world, only when their frequencies match or in other words the rapport is established. Physician should be skilled enough to make the patient forget that he is being interviewed. Dr. Pierre Schmidt once remarked that, "If you are able to make the patient weep or laugh during the first consultation, you have won him and he will stay with you as a very faithful patient." He has thus in a single line summarized what is meant by the term 'rapport' and effective communication.

Homeopathic case taking is all about the art of communication. Effective communication and patient listening are the two sides of the same coin. Effective communication can only result from patient listening and is the first step towards tuning in to somebody. Terms like communication gap are almost always the result of poor listening. Concentration, attentiveness, and avoiding the temptation to interrupt are the keys to skilled listening. Physician should concentrate on 'How it is said'? rather than what is said, as it will allow him to understand the intensity and the type of sensation experienced by the patient. A positive body language is complimentary and essential part of good listening. To enhance the effect of communication physician must enhance body language. According to experts it forms as high as 60% of communication. Dr. Stuart Close stresses on the calm, dignified and patient manner while communicating with the patient. Physician should have an agreeable, pleasant expression and use all possible gestures like nodding yes that encourage the patient to go on with his story of sufferings. He should signal attentiveness by words like 'I see', 'I understand', 'yes.' Such words make the patient feel that the physician is with him throughout the narrative.

Regular eye contact while listening is also important as it makes the patient feel bonded with the conversation. But eye contact does not mean staring.

Interrupting the patient should be strictly avoided. Only if the patient leaves the track then it is essential to bring him back. Physician should guard himself against 'prejudgment', which means judging the remedy while conducting inquiry. During the process of inquiry physician should concentrate on it and he should be unifocal, the activity of conducting inquiry and searching for simillimum should not be mixed up. This is exactly what constitutes prejudiced observation. Physician should only focus of his thoughts on the patient present in front of him, if he wishes to be an attentive listener. Another thing physician should guard himself against is putting questions on 'remedy lines.' Putting words into patient's mouth is a crime in homeopathic interrogation, which all stalwarts have repeatedly warned. Inspite of this even the best physicians cannot resist the temptation of asking leading questions.

The one who wishes to be a good prescriber should constantly check oneself and should constantly prevent oneself from falling into the easy trap of suggestive questions. During the interview when the patient stops narrating, the physician should ask, "what else"? The aim is to drain the patient dry of what he knows about himself. If the patient is talkative the practitioner should prevent him from irrelevant talk. Considerable amount of tact is needed in keeping such patients on main track.

It is an old saying that, "Face is the mirror of emotions." An alert physician should therefore never miss the changes in facial expressions of the patient while describing a complaint. Much can be deduced from watching expressions, movement and gestures. Every face is a reflection of an individual, a unique entity.

Some patients use medical terms while telling their complaints, for example, a patient may say that " I have migraine" or " I have acidity problem" or "I have infection"; in such a case the physician should not ridicule him or her, instead the physician should gently discourage him and ask him to describe, what exactly does he feel? Or what troubles him? Patient should be encouraged to talk and discuss about himself however insignificant it may seem to him.

Time factor should always be kept in mind while conducting the interview, as too long clinical interview proves taxing to the patient and also for those in waiting. An interview should never

Secrets of Effective Case-taking

exceed beyond one hour, otherwise the patient may get restless and would answer to 'Please the doctor.' Real information is lost in such a case. Instead the physician should try to develop the ability to get the vital facts about the case within a limited space of time.

Writing down notes while the patient is describing the emotional side of the story is the last thing to do. It is seen that if it is done the patient suddenly stops or cuts short his description, because he doesn't want his innermost feelings to be noted down and made a record of, which anybody can read, in spite of the fact that he is sure of the privacy of the interview. A patient in most of the cases keeps his real self well hidden although he may seem to be telling everything about himself. But usually even a detailed narration of the patient is just like a film in which he features either as a victim or the hero, but just before leaving the consulting room he may 'spill some beans.' In these moments the patient utters

---

TIPS FOR RAPPORT BUILDING & EFFECTIVE COMMUNICATION

Always:
- Welcome the patient with a smile.
- Make him feel he is important.
- Respect his opinions although you may disagree.
- Make him feel he/she is heard and understood.
- Put yourself in patient's shoes to feel what he feels.
- Try to give true & polite answers to his/her queries.

Never:
- Ridicule a patient if he uses medical terms.
- Show anger & rudeness during conversation.
- Interrupt the patient when he is describing his complaints.
- See your wrist watch when the patient is talking to you.
- Criticize the other physician in front of your patient.
- Make him wait too long in your waiting room.

some sentences, which are the most important facts about him, and these are the sentences, that he wishes he should not have said. These are the words, which slip out from the thick wall he had built to guard himself. It is most likely that he will get irritated if the physician asks him to clarify them.

Investigating the mental side of the case is the trickiest part of homeopathic clinical interview. P. Sankaran has made some useful suggestions in this regard. He states, "At times the patient may try to hide or refuse to reveal some emotional factor. It may be some tragic episode or one which may have an element of personal shame. Then I explain to him that the more he feels like hiding it the more important it is for us, as it will help us to find his remedy. This always brings out his cooperation." He further adds, "In trying to discover the mental or emotional makeup and in uncovering the inner conflicts of the patients, it is always advisable to see the patient alone. Very often there are thoughts and feelings in the mind of the patient which may be unknown even to their closest relatives and which they may never reveal in the presence of anyone else."

Case taking is the art of making patient talk, and making him come out of his shell. A skilled physician makes patient reveal his most closely guarded secrets and his true personality to the physician. Dr. M. L. Dhawale has rightly said that investigation of the life and living style of any individual is a tricky business. We never know enough of it. It is an art, which evolves steadily in a physician motivated in right manner.

FIVE KEY ASPECTS OF CLINICAL INTERVIEW

Five main factors play a major role in homeopathic clinical interview. They are as follows:
1. The consulting room / chamber.
2. Physician's attitude and behaviour.

3. Listening.
4. Questioning.
5. Recording.

The guidelines for clinical interview given by various homeopathic stalwarts mainly revolve around these factors. Majority of guidelines although similar in content, vary a bit in certain aspects. A synopsis of suggestions in the above areas, made by homeopathic masters is presented here with addition of some useful practical tips.

1. THE CONSULTING ROOM / CHAMBER

The atmosphere of the consulting room is an important factor in a clinical interview. Few facts must be kept in mind while planning a consulting room which are as follows:

- A neat and clean consulting room creates a good impression.
- A patient would not reveal his story in an environment that is uncomfortable for him.
- A quiet environment and privacy is must. The consulting chamber should be sound proof for privacy.
- The room should not feel too clinical or formal.
- If the physician is practicing at home, the doors opening into other rooms should be closed.
- The physician should instruct the family members not to disturb him during the case taking.
- In a home based practice, the cooking odours, children making noise, and continuous ringing of doorbell and phone are the things likely to create a disturbance and thus break the link in the interview. The physician should be aware of them. He should try to avoid such disturbances.

- The room should have sufficient light and ventilation.
- The sitting arrangement should be comfortable.
- The patients want to be assured that their details will remain confidential.

2. PHYSICIAN'S ATTITUDE AND BEHAVIOUR

Physician's attitude and behaviour rules the interview more than anything else. Hence one should be fully aware of the type of attitude and behaviour expected of a homeopath during the clinical interview. Following things are necessary in this respect:

- Physician's mind should be free from preoccupation with his own personal problems. *("He should start the case taking with 'blank' paper and 'blank' mind." -P. Sankaran.).*
- He should not conduct the case taking when he himself is emotionally upset or physically ill (having some physical complaint such as headache.)
- All his thoughts should be focused upon the case in hand.
- Homeopathic interview demands the practitioner to be alert, clear minded, free from prejudices and having sound senses.
- He should start the case taking without any preconceived notions about the case.
- He should avoid thinking on remedy lines or feeling that he has seen a similar case earlier.
- The doctor should preferably begin the session with some small talk with the patient instead of directly getting to the questions. This will make the patient comfortable and help in establishing rapport.
- In the beginning the doctor should give an outline of the clinical session. The more one keeps his patient informed the more comfortable the patient gets and thus nothing would surprise him.

Secrets of Effective Case-taking 69

- He can add humour in the conversation to make the patient comfortable.
- The doctor should have a non-judgemental and neutral attitude to whatever the patient is telling.
- He should avoid a formal attitude and be friendly.
- The physician should have the ability to make his patient forget that he is under examination.
- Physician should respect patient's feelings. He should avoid indulging in confrontation or argument with the patient.
- The dignity of the patient should be maintained at any cost.
- The doctor should be calm, dignified and cheerful during interview. He should adapt himself quickly to patient's mood and personality.
- Laughing at the patient, correcting his errors and criticizing him are some of the mannerless behaviours on the part of the physician. They should be strictly avoided.
- He should not show impatience. The doctor should make his patient feel that he has all the time in the world for him.
- He should never appear bored, inattentive, impatient and disinterested during clinical interview.
- Gazing at the window or continually writing notes will put off the patient.
- Eye contact with the patient is necessary during the conversation but gazing fixedly at him should be strictly avoided. If it is done, patient is likely to get anxious and forget what he is narrating.
- The doctor should make it clear from his gestures and expression that he has whole attention to whatever the

patient is telling and that he will not be shocked or angered by anything the patient says or asks.

- The crux of physician's behaviour during case taking lies in an attitude of "watchful expectancy" and "masterly inactivity" (P. Sankaran).

3. LISTENING

Listening forms almost 60% of conversation and hence it is a key factor in homeopathic clinical interview. Following tips must be borne in mind regarding this aspect:

- One should never interrupt his patient while he is telling his story.
- Attentive listening can really help a doctor to tune into the patient and establish a basis for solid communication.
- Alert mind and concentration are must for attentive listening.
- Attentive listening encourages the patient to continue with his narration.
- The doctor should consciously avoid getting distracted by exterior 'noises' while listening.
- He should not get distracted by his own concerns or thoughts about what he is going to do or say next, while listening.
- While listening, the physician should also pay attention to patient's body language i.e. his posture, his appearance and expressions and tone of voice, etc. This may reveal to him the intensity of the complaints felt by the patient. Many other things also get expressed through body language.
- Doctor should concentrate on how it is said rather than what is said. This makes him able to read the signs; the

- body language, speech patterns and rhythms, levels of apparent tension or calmness add to the meaning of what the patient is saying.
- While listening, the doctor should also take note of nonverbal hints and hidden meanings.
- Physician's facial expressions should be such that the patient feels that the doctor is interested in whatever the patient is telling.
- Gestures like chin resting in fisted hand, nodding of head with concentrated expression, etc. give an impression that doctor is listening attentively. This type of body language is good from the point of view of active listening.
- Attentive listening should be continued until the patient comes to a full stop.

4. QUESTIONING

Questioning is an art that develops during the course of practice. The quality of information obtained during clinical interview largely depends upon the way in which questions are framed. However, some useful tips must be kept in mind while interrogating the patient:

- Questions should be put in simple words.
- Physician should try to complete each symptom with respect to location, sensations, modalities, concomitants and causation by putting specific questions if some symptoms are incomplete.
- Questions are asked to clarify certain points and to complete the information that has been already given.
- While questioning the practitioner should restrict himself to one symptom or area at a time. Patients get confused when questioned about 2/3 different symptoms or areas at a time.

- Do not use technical language or English while questioning. It is better to be acquainted with local language of the place where one is practicing as it helps in putting questions that the patients easily understand.
- Physician should make sure that the patient understands his questions and he understands patient's answers and queries.
- Physician must make sure that he has questioned the patient on every system and function. If this is not done the important details might get missed out.
- Do not put same question twice as the patient might think that the physician is inattentive.
- Putting the same question in a different context and by changing the wording is sometimes required to assess the patient. The replies received determine the extent to which the patient is a reliable observer.
- Specific questions are sometimes necessary when definite information seems missing inspite of best efforts.
- Questions that interrupt patient's chain of thought and make him go away from the point he is narrating must be avoided.
- Physician should avoid skipping questioning on sexual sphere due to modesty. Tact is required while questioning on sexual aspect. It should be done without making the patient feel embarrassed in the process. If the physician explains the importance of inquiry in sexual sphere right in the beginning of the interview, the patient would not hesitate to give information in this important area.
- **While investigating patient's mind the questions should be such that they do not hurt the patient's feelings directly and are easy to understand.**

Secrets of Effective Case-taking

- Patients do not give much information when directly asked about mental sphere. Hence, questions that help in knowing the life events such as illnesses suffered, type of parents, type of siblings, type of relatives, family and work environment and school experiences, etc. need to be asked to know patient's mental state.

> **Key rules are:**
> Avoid direct questions.
> Avoid leading questions.
> Avoid questions along remedy lines.
> Avoid questions that suggest answers.
> Avoid questions with multiple-choice answers.
> Avoid insinuating or accusing type questions.

5. RECORDING

Proper recording of whatever is narrated by the patient is necessary. A properly recorded case goes a long way in helping the physician in determining the similar remedy. The tips are as follows:

- The format of case taking should be ready before one begins to take the case.
- Physician should be in the habit of writing faster as some patients narrate their sufferings with great speed and spontaneously.
- A homeopath should be able to record the symptoms simultaneously while questioning or communicating with the patient.
- Information obtained should be recorded in patient's own words.
- One should start each symptom with fresh line.

- Practitioner should not forget to record the intensities of sensations experienced and modalities.
- The history of patient's previous illnesses should be recorded in chronological order. The nature of symptoms, duration, severity and treatment received earlier should also be recorded.
- Information about patient's general appearance, skin colour, facial expressions, way of sitting, posture and gait, etc. also needs to be recorded along with whatever patient narrates.

INQUIRY IN PEDIATRIC CASES

Inquiry in case of children varies from that conducted in case of adults. Apart from the regular heads of inquiry certain other areas relevant in case of children need to be investigated. So the format varies from that adopted in other cases. Hence inquiry needs to be done right from the time of conception and therefore involves various headings under which it is to be done and which are necessary for a homeopath. These include mother's gestation notes, developmental milestones, vaccination history, neonatal problems, history of pica, etc.

OBSERVATION AND EXAMINATION OF CHILDREN

- Mother's information.
- Physician's observation.
- Physical examination.
- Avoid observation along remedy lines.
- Developmental milestones.
- Academic performance.
- Reactions.
- Sensitivity.

- Behavioural pattern.
- Eating habits and feeding schedule.
- Vivid description in chronic cases.

Case taking in children requires special skills and training on part of physician because they can't speak for themselves and parent's account dominates the interview. Especially the mother serves as a good source of information. Apart from parents physician's keen observation is required and it is more important in these cases than in any other case. The homeopath must judge the accuracy of the second hand information provided by the parents.

Problem is posed when both the parents lack in observation and are unable to describe more than one or two prominent complaints. In such a case physical examination and observation are the only means of getting the information. Physical examination is more important in acute complaints of infants, because infants know only one way of telling their complaints that is crying. Essence of examining children lies in making them comfortable and gaining their confidence so that they don't cry during physical examination. A padiatrician from Bristol has in one line expressed the essence of physical examination in children, he says that, "If a child cries when you examine it, then it is probably your fault." In acute cases when mother is describing what is wrong with her child the physician should observe the child. The look of his face, his expressions and his movements all should be observed carefully.

A child is quiet when mother is carrying him into the waiting room suddenly starts crying if the mother keeps him on the chair in the consulting room; it may be an indication that he needs *Chamomilla* for his complaints, because it is the *Chamomilla* child who wants to be carried. Whereas a shy child who hides behind mother and does not face the physician is obviously hinting at

'Baryta.' During the course of case taking the mother tells that he frequently takes cold and is grossly deficient in studies, here a co-relation of physician's observation with the information given by the mother would surely fix *Baryta carb.* as the remedy. A child belonging to *Antimony* type would cry out loud if the physician looks at him, touches him and tries to feel his pulse, he hates it. There are numerous other examples where without even a single question and merely by keen observation of the behaviour and attitude of the child physician gets indications for suitable remedy.

Thus, in paediatric cases *'actions do speak louder than words!'* An observant physician never misses these indications and can even treat those paediatric cases with success, where parents lack observation and information is very scanty. But observation needs to be logically co-related with other available information to be sure of ones prescription.

An alert physician should be cautious to avoid 'observation on remedy lines' as it is this kind of mal-observation and prejudice that Hahnemann wants us to be cautious about.

Preferably both the parents should be present during the interview so that when one parent fails to reply properly the other one comes handy. It is usual to find one of the parents lacking in observation while the other one compensating for it. History of developmental milestones is an important area of inquiry in paediatric cases. If the child is between 4-8 years of age parents tend to forget the approximate months where the child crossed a particular milestone in development. So the questions have to be framed in such a manner that they will refresh their memories. Take for example the question, how much did he talk on his first birthday? Or had his late walking or talking been a matter of worry, that time? In both these questions, it is likely that the parents would remember the month as most of the parents are sensitive to delays in their child's growth and they have a sentimental value attached to it. Therefore, questions framed in the above manner can most of the times yield quick answers.

When inquired about the child's academic performance most of the parents avoid referring to their child's poor studies. Considering this, cross-examination becomes necessary and here questions such as, if he is good in studies then why he needs tuitions need to be asked, and questions such as what do his teachers tell about his studies and his behaviour in school? Have you received any complaints regarding his behaviour in school from the teachers. Questions like these help the physician to access the child's interaction in school environment and his inclination to studies. Inquiry regarding reaction to strangers, reaction to physical pain, reaction to punishment or being rebuked and reaction to arrival of new sibling, and reaction to death in family also provides valuable information. Sensitivity to parents fighting, to movies, to horror stories, to tensions in family, are also important facets of inquiry in case of children. They help the physician in knowing the mind (mentals) of the child.

Behavioural pattern varies from one child to another child, and needs to be investigated through proper questioning because that is what differentiates one child from another child and one remedy from another in homeopathic materia medica too. Another thing to keep in mind is that, if the child is old enough to express and intervenes in the conversation he should be allowed to talk. Physician should not be averse to any information just because it is coming from the child; he should be encouraged to tell more.

Faulty eating habits, poor appetite and overfeeding can be interpreted from inquiring about the number of times the child eats and about feeding schedule in infants. This will also shed light on the child's cravings and aversions. If any disproportion is noticed in quantity and type of intake the physician can advise the parents about faulty feeding in infants and regarding the dietary precautions in older children.

Sometimes in a chronic case, parents describe the child's complaints in vague terms due to long interval between two episodes of acute attack, or exacerbations, in such cases the parents should be asked to visualize or remember what had happened at 'that time,' so that the whole scene of illness comes to their mind and then they are able to describe well.

PHYSICAL EXAMINATION

Essential components are:
- Gain patient's confidence.
- Diagnosis.
- Prognosis.
- Prevention.
- Selection of cases.
- Environment.
- Privacy.

Secondary importance of physical examination consequent upon the secondary importance of diagnosis in homeopathy is well known. In most of the cases the novice is under the impression that a clinical interview will suffice to provide him the information he needs. As a result many physicians since the time of Hahnemann have neglected it. It is surprising that we can still find homeopathic clinics without examination table and other instruments like stethoscope and B.P. apparatus, which are necessary for examination.

Physical examination is a must and complementary to the procedure of case taking. In fact, physical examination has many concealed advantages that we cannot afford to overlook. A thorough and gentle examination is often reassuring to the patient. The gentle touch that the patient experiences conveys many things without saying a single word. There lies an inherent power of communication in touching the patient. It conveys to the patient that the doctor is with him; the doctor cares for him and also conveys the warmth of the physician, which can never be expressed in words. It plays an important role in gaining patient's confidence.

The physical examination should be carried out at the end in homeopathic consultation because if carried out in the beginning it will highlight the diagnostic aspect of treatment that would naturally lead to hindrances in acquiring the information necessary for a homeopath. Physical examination; helps the physician in establishing diagnosis after examination only the physician is in a position to answer all the queries regarding what the future holds for the patient with regard to his disease and the precautions that the patient is expected to take. It will also help the physician in selection of cases, which is a must in homeopathic practice. Sometimes a life threatening condition may go unnoticed if the physician has not examined the patient and if this happens it may prove hazardous to physician's reputation.

As for instances a large tumour may go unnoticed, as there is no pain, or what is considered to be a case of piles might turnout to be a case of rectal tumor or growth after physical examination or in some cases the patient comes with some trivial complaints but on measuring his blood pressure is found to be very high; here quick measures to bring it to normal are necessary to avoid complications. Thus, the seriousness of the disease can only be determined by thorough physical examination.

Physical examination is a must to avoid pitfalls in practice; this should be always kept in mind. According to Sir Robert Hutchinson, a good physical examination requires a co-operative patient and a quiet, warm and well-lit room. Daylight is better than artificial light because the latter may mask changes in skin colour, for example the faint yellow tinge of slight jaundice. Although in practice the examination may have to be made under all sorts of circumstances, every attempt should be made to reassure and relax the patient.

In case of the physical examination of a female patient especially when a male doctor is examining a female patient and where the examination involves private organs, the precaution to be taken is that a female attendant or the mother or whosoever accompanies the patient should be present in the room during the examination. This is done to reassure the patient and to protect the physician from subsequent accusations of improper conduct. In gynecological cases it is sometimes better to refer the patient to gynaecologist for physical examination and opinion before starting the homeopathic treatment.

DOCUMENTATION IN HOMEOPATHIC PRACTICE (THE CASE RECORD)

Importance of maintaining case records in homeopathic practice is a well known truth. One must be fully aware of the 'Why' and 'How' of homeopathic documentation. In this respect 'Why' deals with reasons for maintaining a case record, while the 'How' deals with the method of keeping records and noting down information.

Dr. Boenninghausen considered case records indispensable to every true homeopath. He was of the view that physician's memory cannot store all the facts about all the cases even if the practice is moderately extended one; hence record keeping is a must for a homeopath. Some physicians are unfortunately very negligent about this aspect of homeopathic practice. They consider jotting down changes in patient's symptoms and medicines prescribed as maintaining case records. Instead a well-maintained case record incorporates, a well taken case, reports of investigations carried out by the patient, record of medicines (both allopathic as well as homeopathic) he has taken earlier, and the physician's observations with date notes on changes in symptoms and prescriptions made by the physician from time to time. A standardized case record format has to be followed. The proforma of case taking *(See Appendix A)* may vary from physician to physician but the best and experienced homeopaths seem to follow a similar outline with little variations. The proforma should not be out of tune with the one followed by majority of expert physicians.

Mentioning the intensities of symptoms while recording the case is an important part of homeopathic documentation. Numerical system of recording the intensity is easy to adopt. Failure to note down the intensities of various symptoms i.e. pain 3, stiffness 3, anger 3, etc. would lead to a flat case record, which is of little help in individualisation. Consideration of intensity is important in establishing similarity between the patient and the remedy. But one should be very careful while giving intensities to the symptoms only the symptoms; which are spontaneously narrated by the patient and which are intensely felt and which are clearly narrated, not open to two interpretations should be given intensity. This is must to avoid prejudice in giving intensities. The striking and strange symptoms should be underlined. Symptoms recorded in patient's words should be denoted with single inverted commas for example, 'My head feels blocked', 'I feel as if there is a ball in my stomach.' From the day one of homeopathic practice the number of case records grows steadily but surely, therefore, a suitable indexing and numbering system should be developed by individual physician as per his requirements. This will prevent wastage of time and waiting period of the patient would be minimised, as the case record will be found within no time. Handing over the case record to the patient should be totally avoided, as it may get lost or spoiled and in such a situation the doctor is in total dark when the patient visits him next time. Well-maintained case record has multiple advantages.

In aphorism 104 of Organon, Hahnemann stresses the utility of maintaining case-record. He calls it a guide to physician in his treatment. Here he also describes the procedure that is to be followed whenever the patient visits the physician next time. To put it in his words, "At this fresh examination of the patient he only needs to strike out of the list of symptoms noted down at the first visit those that have become ameliorated, to mark what still remain and add any new symptoms that may have supervened." Apart from what has been suggested by Hahnemann, another way to record the symptoms in follow-up is to put > sign in front of the symptoms which have ameliorated. For e.g. itching > or burning in rectum >, etc. The degree of amelioration can be denoted as > 2 or > 3 depending upon correct judgement of patient's description. The symptoms that are not ameliorated can be denoted by + sign i.e. pain + or sneezing +. While underlining each one of them can denote new symptoms.

Apart from serving as a guide to the physician the case records also serve as a teaching and training material for clinical training of future generation of homeopaths. Case records of well-treated cases in possession of a physician speak volumes about his failures and successes. The mechanism of action of our drugs being quite nebulous, hence the results are only yardstick in our work. Thus the record of well treated and cured cases are much useful to demonstrate the efficiency of homeopathy.

The introduction of computers in homeopathy has made the homeopathic documentation more systematic and easily accessible. The number of homeopaths having computers is increasing day by day. If all the practitioners having computers maintain systematic case records, it would definitely help the homeopathic fraternity worldwide. Collected data from various individuals (homeopaths) can be stored in one computer and processed further. This will help in using the case records for education and research for the coming generation of homeopaths.

Speaking with passion but without facts is like making a beautiful dive into an empty pool; forgetting this dictum homeopathic lecturers, physicians and those who address various

Secrets of Effective Case-taking 83

seminars and conferences, and physicians claiming cures in homeopathic journals coat cases from their practice and make claims but these claims need to be verified by way of well kept records, but till now this has been totally overlooked by homeopaths and students in general. A physician making tall claims is never questioned with regards to evidences and records to logically support his claims of being a scientific homeopath. Boenninghausen had rightly said that the records are useful to satisfy legal requirement for possible future defence, the demand for which may be expected. This is true especially in the present times, considering the fact that medical services have been covered under the Consumer Protection Act.

PROFORMA OF CASE TAKING

It is very important to have an outline or schema of case-taking handy before one proceeds to take the case. A standardized case taking proforma often makes the task easier for the treating physician. The format of case taking adopted by various physicians and educational institutions differ in certain aspects. There is no standardized pattern of case taking that is accepted by one and all till today. An effort to standardize the case record is made by Institute of Clinical Research (ICR), Mumbai. Based on Standardized Case Record better known as SCR of ICR, a proforma of case taking is given in *Appendix A* so as to aid the homeopath in taking the case, hoping that the careful reader will take full advantage of the proforma. *(Note: SCR is adopted by Central Council of Research in Homeopathy. The SCR has been used by ICR since 1975 in all its educational programmes most successfully.)*

Appendix B shows the format of recording follow up responses of the patient, whereas *Appendix C* shows the Case Index Card to be given to the patient so as to make the retrieval of the case paper easy on the patient's follow up visit.

APPENDIX A

PROFORMA OF CASE TAKING

Name: Case Index No.:

Age: Sex: Date:

Education:

Occupation:

Marital Status: Single/Married/Widow/Divorce

Habit: Veg/Non-veg/Eggs

Religion/Caste:_____

Residential Address:

Phone No.:   Email:

Referred by:

PRESENT HISTORY

I. Chief Complaint

LOCATION	SENSATION	MODALITIES	CONCOMITANTS
Area, Direction and Pathology Spread, Tissue Organ, System & Duration		A.F. & < >	(Strict time relation)

II. Associated Complaints

1. LOCATION   SENSATION   MODALITIES   CONCOMITANTS

2. LOCATION   SENSATION   MODALITIES   CONCOMITANTS

III. Patient as a Person

General Appearance: (Body built, Complexion, Facial expression, Carriage & Gait)

Height: Weight:

Physician's Observations:

Appetite: Thirst:

Cravings:

Aversions:

Disordered by:

Addictions/
Pica (in infants & children):

Natural Eliminations

Stool (Character, Frequency, Satisfaction, Urging, Complaints - Before / During / After)

Urine (Colour, Odour, Frequency, Complaints - Before/During/After)

Perspiration (Quantity, Stains, Parts, Odour)

Sleep and Dreams

Duration:

Character: Deep / Refreshing / Unrefreshing / Poor / Siesta / Disturbed

Complaints (Before / During / After sleep, related to sleep)

Dreams:

Sex Function

Desire: Moderate / Increased / Diminished (Recent Deviations)

Sex: Marital / Premarital / Extramarital

Frequency:

Habits:
Complaints (During Coition, After Coition):

Menstrual Function

FMP (first menstrual period):

LMP (last menstrual period):

Frequency:

Duration:

Quantity:

Modalities:

Character (Colour & appearance):

Stains: Fast/ Washable   Odour:

Complaints (Before Menses, During Menses, After Menses)

Leucorrhoea

(Character, Occurrence, Modalities)

History of Pregnancies and Abortions

Pregnancies

Gravida: Para:

Abortions: Normal / Induced / Habitual / Threatened

(Following information is required for Paediatric Cases)

Mother's Gestation Notes

Pregnancy: Wanted/ Unwanted

Foetal movements:

Delivery Type: F.T.N.D. (Full term normal delivery), Caesar, Episotomy done

Forceps   Premature

Antenatal History

Mental State/Complaints during Pregnancy:

Physical Complaints during Pregnancy:

Drugs:

Lochia: Lactation:

Neonatal problems: Birth weight:

Secrets of Effective Case-taking

Developmental milestones

Head holding:

Turning in bed:

Crawling:

Teething:

Sitting with support:

Sitting without support:

Monosyllables:

True speech (sentences):

Walking with support:

Walking without support:

Anterior fontanalle:

Posterior fontanalle:

Feeding Schedule:

Vaccination History:

Life Space

(This includes a clear-cut picture of patient's relationships with family members, friends and associations. Family includes those relatives living with the patient as well as separately. Trace the picture backwards to childhood and forward to the present time. Patient's emotional nature, intellectual attainments and aspirations. Emotions relate to patient's feelings such as anger, sadness, love, hate, fear, fright, anxiety, etc. Intellectual attainments relate to patient's perception, memory, ideas, awareness, discrimination judgement, motivation as well as performance in different situations such as work, family, and society.)

Physical Reactions

Bathing:

Fanning:

Covers:

Food & drink:

Cold drinks:

Season: Winter: Summer: Rainy:

Change of weather/temp./season: Wet getting:

Heat of sun: Warm room:

Moist air/A.C./Cooler: Thunderstorm :

Cloudy weather: Cold damp weather:

Type of clothing preferred:

PAST HISTORY

FAMILY HISTORY

Father: Mother:

PGM   MGM
(Paternal Grandmother)   (Maternal Grandmother)

PGF: MGF:
(Paternal Grandfather)   (Maternal Grandfather)

Paternal Uncles: Maternal Uncles:

Paternal Aunts: Maternal Aunts:

PHYSICAL EXAMINATION

Temperature: Pulse:

Blood Pressure:

Conjunctiva: Nails:

Tongue: Skin:

Lymph nodes (Glands):   Throat:

Systemic Examination

Respiratory System:

CVS:

P/A:

INVESTIGATIONS DONE

Provisional Diagnosis & Clinical Diagnosis:

Remarks :

PLANNING OF TREATMENT

Remedy Selected:
(with Potency and Repetition)
(Acute, Chronic, Intercurrent & Constitutional)

Follow-up with Prescription:

APPENDIX B

FORMAT OF FOLLOW-UP

Date	Notes	Prescription

APPENDIX C

SPECIMEN OF CASE INDEX CARD

Dr. Deshmukh's Homeopathic Clinic
Name:_____
Age:_____ Sex:_____ Date:_____
Diagnosis:_____
Case Index Number:
Please bring this card on your next visit.

CHAPTER 5

KNOWING PATIENT'S 'PSYCHE': A SYSTEMATIC APPROACH

- ❖ The mental state   99
- ❖ Prerequisites for perceiving mental state 101
- ❖ What to ask?   101
- ❖ Interpreting patient's story   104
- ❖ Illustrative case I   107
- ❖ Illustrative case II   117
- ❖ A case for working   131

CHAPTER 5

KNOWING PATIENT'S 'PSYCHE': A SYSTEMATIC APPROACH

The fundamental philosophy of homeopathy stresses on knowing the patient as a person. A homoeopath is expected to understand the 'Man' who is ill rather than the illness itself. Speedy recovery and cure is guaranteed if he is able to match this man with the most closely resembling image in the materia medica. But what does the 'man' consist of? Well, the obvious answer would be mind and body. Body is gross. It follows certain natural laws. Body can be known by how it appears and by it's qualities in any field of action. Mind is subtle. It does not follow natural laws. It is not bound by time. It is difficult to understand or comprehend mind due to its timelessness. Therefore, for centuries mind remains an unsolved puzzle. If we turn to history of medical science we find that doctors recognised the role of 'Psyche' or 'Mind' in illness, but their treatment was concerned more with body than mind and to some extent this type of practice still continues. However, as the knowledge evolved physicians realised that mind had a definite role to play in genesis and maintenance of disease, hence ardent study began and soon it was realised that when mind was affected body was affected concomitantly. Mind as a causative factor came to light and thus came the concept of psychosomatic diseases. Modern medicine started to recognise the causative aspect of mind.

Kent believed that mind gets affected first and then everything else is affected. He termed bacteria only as scavengers of disease. He relegated all diseases to mind. According to him, diseases travelled only in one direction, that is, from mind to body. After Kent, Boger gave equal importance to both mind and body in his work. He was of the view that the mind and body together by their interplay are causing disease.

The mind and body by their interplay cause the phenomenon of disease; in illness both mind and body play a role. Doctors must study both. If they only focus on physical aspect and do not pay attention to patient's psyche they would fail miserably in treating the patient as a whole. Hahnemann realised this fact and hence devoted 20 aphorisms of his monumental work Organon to mind. In these 20 paragraphs he talked of mental symptoms and he discussed following different varieties of mental diseases:

1. Diseases which started in mind and remained in mind.
2. Diseases that started at physical level and over a period of time mind got affected.
3. Diseases that started at mental level and descended to physical level.

In aphorism 210 Hahnemann writes, '*... and in all cases of disease we are called on to cure the state of patient's disposition is to be particularly noted, along with the totality of the symptoms, if we would trace an accurate picture of the disease in order to be able therefrom to treat it homoeopathically with success.*'

Hahnemann asks a homeopath to take note of the state of patient's disposition, which means he wants that a homeopath should note patient's state of mind, that is, mental state. Hence, to know patient's 'Psyhe' or mental state one must be very clear with regards to what does it consist of and only then one is in a position to know a patient's mental state or mind.

THE MENTAL STATE

It is important to note that mental symptoms and mental state are two different things. The mental state is an abstraction which is derived from the peripheral data (symptoms). Mental symptoms furnish us with only a partial evidence of the deeper underlying mental state. The individuals mental state has to be perceived or conceived from whatever observation the physician can make of the patient's 'actions' that is, his behaviour and his responses. Various expressions like weeping etc. as seen through patient's behaviour are the only evidence of mental state which is not something material. The patient's mental state has to be interpreted by observing and understanding why and how of his responses or reactions to various situations in his life, in the areas of work, family and society. His responses in different phases of life (childhood, adolescence, adulthood etc.) need to be interpreted in an unprejudiced manner to arrive at his 'Psyche', 'mind' or 'mental state.' The mental state is a dynamic resultant of an individual's responses to the environmental stimuli (or situations) which affect him.

The responses or reactions to various situations which get repeated over a period constitute the 'mental state.' It consists of certain basic attributes or traits of an individual. The basic attributes of a patient's mind categorized under following headings:

- Intellect
- Emotions
- Behaviour
- Functioning

Intellect includes:

Capacities

- Perception
- Ideation
- Thinking
- Decision making
- Confidence
- Judgement

Performance (which depends upon motivation and will)

Emotions include:

- Anger
- Sadness
- Envy
- Jealousy
- Fear
- Fright
- Anxiety etc.

It is this mental state which Hahnemann wants us to match with that of a homeopathic remedy. He writes in aphorism 213 of 'Organon' *'....if we do not, in every case of disease, even in such as are acute, observe, along with the other symptoms, those relating to the changes in the state of the mind and disposition and if we do not select, for the patient's relief, from among the medicines a disease-force which, in addition to the similarity of its other symptoms to those of the disease, is also capable of producing a similar state of the disposition and mind.'*

PREREQUISITES FOR PERCEIVING MENTAL STATE

WHAT IS DEMANDED FROM A PHYSICIAN TO PERCEIVE PATIENT'S MENTAL STATE ACCURATELY?

Dr M.L. Dhawale writes, 'The physician requires to be sensitive at all levels, must learn to vibrate with the patient at the level of feelings while maintaining his intellectual discipline and poise which give him the requisite discrimination to arrive at proper judgements in respect of the troubles narrated by the patient.'

'The physician must be a master of the interview technique and capable of dealing with all types of patients. He must be able to plan the interview in the first few minutes of contact with the patient and program it as demanded by the situation as it changes from time to time. This demands versatility in operations.'

'He must have the competence to relate the mental state to the total experience of the patient in his setting. When he does that, he has erected the Hahnemannian Integrated Totality which can, now, guide him to the simillimum, provided he is also a master at the repertorial technique and a good student of the source books of the homeopathic materia medica.'

WHAT TO ASK?

During the case-taking, physician tries to understand the patient as a person and tries to find out what has lead to his illness. The aim of case taking is to find out the nature of problems faced by the patient, understanding his expectations, his responses to environment, failures and satisfactions so that his mental state can be interpreted.

But patient's mental state cannot be comprehended unless the physician gathers detailed information about him. Getting all the data required to know the patient's mind is a difficult and tricky business. What to ask is the million-dollar question. Direct questioning would not yield anything. Hence, prior to the clinical interview (case-taking) a patient should be asked to write a detailed account of his life till now, that is, his life story from childhood till the present time. He should be asked to write (prior to the interview) or tell (during the interview) the different situations he or she has come across in his or her life and how he or she reacted to them in various phases of life. Patient should be asked to write or tell his memories in three different areas, that is, work, family and society. He should be asked to talk about himself, his nature, hobbies, activities, his likes, his loves and hates, and changes in his nature in the recent past that he or she has observed. A chronology of important events and epochs in patient's life must be there. He or she should be asked to write or describe the important persons (living and dead) associated with him or her from birth till the day in various areas of life (work, family and society). Patient's interpersonal relationships must be inquired in to because many a times a patient's mental or physical problems take birth from his disturbed relationships in the family and /or work situations. A report of patient's nature and behaviour needs to be collected from his close family members too. However, if we ask the close relatives they are most likely to add their own colours and therefore the information gathered from them must be sieved.

A physician should not forget to take note of patient's physical appearance, mode of dressing, his non-verbal mannerisms, body language and frequently repeated words or sentences and typical verbal expressions etc. Patient's behaviour felt or observed during case taking should also be noted.

The key points of inquiry in various important areas can be summarized as follows:

WORK

Nature and type: Present occupation/job/profession/business.

History: Of previous jobs in chronological order, reasons for leaving earlier jobs and/or businesses.

Expectations from patient: Of parents and teacher (if a student), working hours, type of stresses and strains, difficulties faced in carrying out occupational responsibilities.

Performance: Number of promotions, achievements (of targets), profit or losses in business, marks or percentage (if a student), biggest failures and biggest successes, failures if any and the causes of failures. Fear of failure and what patient felt after he failed (reaction to failure)

Interpersonal relations: With boss and subordinates, work sharing help taken or given etc. with teachers (if a student) and with customers (if a businessperson or shopkeeper).

Work: Aims and ambition, satisfaction, aversion to, excess, efficiency, confidence level while performing the job, decision-making abilities and mental or physical fatigue.

FAMILY

- **Type:** Nuclear or joint family set up. Details of people who are living with patient needs to be taken.
- **History:** Childhood home environment, history of quarrels and/or disputes and difference of opinion with family members and among family members, patient's response to their disputes. Grief from loss of close family member or members. Difference in the relationship with parents before and after marriage, difficulties in adapting to 'in laws' faced during initial adjustment period after marriage, type of marriage (love or arranged) and details of each marriage if patient is married more than one time.
- **Interpersonal relations:** With father, mother, siblings, wife, or husband, father in law, mother in law, cousins, uncles and aunts.

- **Attachment:** Most attached to whom and why? Relative most loved or hated by patient and reason for it?
- What is the opinion of close family members about him? (about his nature)
- Patient's opinion about the nature and behaviour of other family members towards him?

SOCIETY

- **Nature and type:** Of current social contacts, membership of any club, association society or political party, posts held in any such organization and activities carried out.
- Social work with any NGO (Non-government organization). Mixing with neighbours and participation in social programmes. Socio-economic setup of area or colony where patient resides.
- **History:** Of disputes with friends and neighbours. Any friend or neighbour with whom patient has totally cut his contacts or relations, if yes then the reason for doing so?
- **Interpersonal relations:** With friends, number of friends, male or female, relations with them, type of friendship, formal/close/very close, with neighbours.
- **Attachment:** With friends/neighbours, most attached to whom and why? Most hated friend/neighbour and cause of hatred.
- Does the patient like company or prefers being alone?
- Is he/she an extrovert or introvert?

All this will give the physician raw material to process in order to identify patient's mental state or to know his personality traits.

INTERPRETING PATIENT'S STORY

Patient's life story needs to be interpreted logically, in an unprejudiced manner, in order to avoid errors in perceiving the mental state. It is easier said then done.

A physician who has a general idea of human behaviour and a general idea of the evolution of mind is in a better position to interpret patient's story to arrive at his basic attributes. A physician will have to keep his own mental 'mirror' as clean as possible because the type of image of the patient's mind depends on the

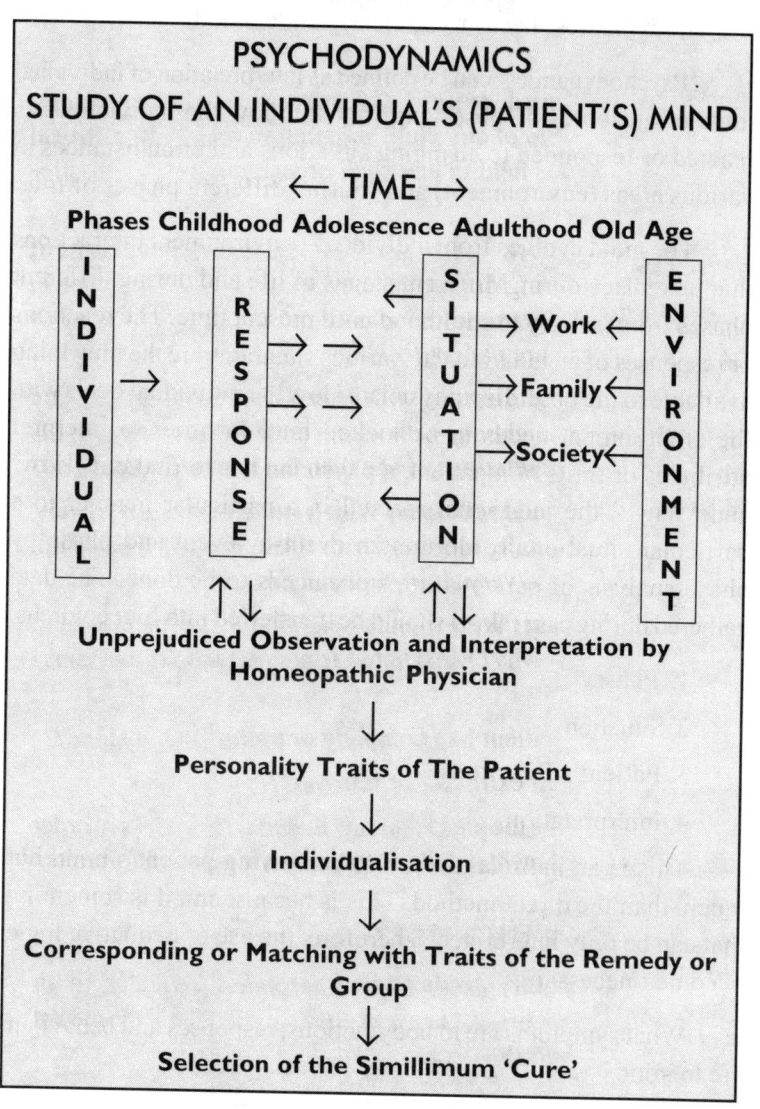

'mirror' (physician) used to form the image. He should avoid (as far as possible) colouring patient's story with his own biases. A 'Psychodynamic Study' of patient's life story needs to be done to arrive at patient's basic mental attributes, so that a suitable remedy with similar mental attributes can be found. What do we mean by 'Psychodynamics' needs to be clearly understood?

'Psychodynamics' can be defined as interpretation of individual traits or attributes by observing why and how the individual has reacted or responded to changing situations and circumstances in various areas (environment) and during different phases of life.

The mind evolves from individual – environment interactions that take place during different stages of life and during different phases from infancy to adulthood until present time. The reactions or responses of an individual to various situations are the only thing available to the observing physician. How the individual deals with the environment needs to be looked into. In order to interpret attributes or traits of a patient, a physician has to find out 'How' and 'Why?' the individual reacted in a particular manner to a particular situation. To do this an event-by-event and phase by phase analysis of patient's life story needs to be done. The data gathered during case taking should be transferred into four columns.

1. Phase
2. Situation
3. Patient's Reactions
4. Interpretation

This is an indirect method of perceiving patient's mind but much than the direct method. This is because mind is something that can be only interpreted. Therefore, the use of deductive logic becomes necessary.

What symptoms are to body, actions, responses and behaviour are to mind.

Patient's mental state is only available to a careful observer of patient's actions and behaviour. It is not something like thirst, appetite or pain, which can be asked about directly. There are no fixed rules neither there are any specific guidelines that can be given regarding interpretation of patient's story. It is something that develops over a period, by repeated exposure to various life stories and their interpretation, provided it is carried out under the guidance of an experienced observer. To facilitate the understanding of how the mental state is interpreted from patient's autobiography, some illustrative cases are given here.

ILLUSTRATIVE CASE I
(Interpreting patient's story)

Name: Mrs. SS **Age:** 28 years
Education: HSC passed in 1995 **Occ.:** Housewife
Marriage: June 2001 **Religion:** Hindu
Habit: Non-vegetarian
Date of birth: 01/04/1977

Chief Complaints

- Recurrent attacks of violent headaches
- Pain in epigastrium
- Acne on face.

Appointment on October 18, 2005.

The data from a thorough clinical interview is as follows:

Describing her childhood she states that, she was the eldest child born in a poor family. Her parents could not afford even milk therefore; she did not get milk after the age of 6 months. She stayed with her parents until the age of 6 years. She has bitter and painful memories of an incident, which occurred when she was 3-4 years old. Mother did not come to pick her up from school, she felt very bad and started crying, she started walking thinking that her home is near by but got lost. An autorikshaw driver picked her up and she stayed with him for 2 days, then he went to police to inform about her, meanwhile her parents also found her with the help of police. She has memories of another childhood incident, which she described. While staying with her parents when she was in 4th standard she was lying on a 'Khat' her father came and pulled her arm and asked her to wash his clothes, she felt very irritated and said she would do it later. She did not keep any verbal communication with her father for next 6 months after this incident. Her father was an irritable person. As she was the eldest amongst siblings, she always fought with her father for the rights of her siblings. As a child, she could not accept denial and wanted whatever she asked for. She must have anything she wanted immediately otherwise she used to cry a lot and create a scene. She was a stubborn child. Her parents could not afford her upbringing and her uncle did not have a child so her uncle brought her up from the age of 6 years. She feels that she was not taken care of well and got less attention at her uncle's place. It would have been much better if she had stayed with her parents. Her uncle used to keep toiletries etc. locked in a cupboard and did not allow her to use or touch it. She felt very sad, got angry and wept a lot.

She got 65% in SSC and never failed. She states she was good in academics until 12th standard but failed in science in 12th standard. During that period, her physics 'tutor' proposed her and she said 'yes' and had an affair with him, wanted to marry him but her uncle opposed it. Her uncle thought she had a bad character and he spoke cheap things about her. She quarreled with her uncle. He had bad intensions about her (in her words 'uncle ki mere par buri nazar thi'). She got very angry and beat up her uncle for making unjust remarks on her character. She hates him and has not seen her uncle's face since that day. Her mother also opposed her love marriage with her physics tutor. Mother was of the opinion that her marriage would adversely affect her siblings' future prospects. She was mentally very upset and did not keep any contacts with him after that. After her failure in 12th, her father stopped supporting her financially, she had strained relations with uncle so could not continue her education. She did odd jobs to earn and helped her sisters financially. She met her present husband while working in a STD booth. He belongs to a lower caste. She married him in June 2001. Since there was a strong opposition from both the families, they did not keep contact with them (patient and her husband). Parents of both sides never visit their home. This makes her feel very sad and lonely. She had once thought that her mother-in-law would be like her mother and she will get care and attention, which she did not get earlier. She was very depressed and used to weep a lot, as there was no one to look after her during her first pregnancy. There was nobody whom she could tell her physical complaints and take help from. Her husband, who is a driver in railways, goes out on duty and she is alone at home. She cannot concentrate on anything. Even while watching television or taking lunch she is constantly thinking, feeling sad and lonely. Feels the absence of elders at home.

DESCRIPTION OF THE PATIENT

Built: Thin and has a dark complexion.

Height: 5ft. 1"

Weight: 40 kg.

Personality: She is angry by nature. If somebody acts against her wishes and passes unjust remarks, she quarrels with that person. If her husband does not bring what she asked for, she gets angry and quarrels with him, weeps a lot. Does not accept the thing if it is brought later. She always takes the right side and stands by the truth but she cannot tolerate lies whenever there is a dispute or altercation. She feels fearful and bad thoughts come to her mind when she is alone in house. She has fear of darkness especially when alone. She never wants to be alone and wants company. Whenever she is hurt, she weeps easily. She starts trembling with anger and wants to beat the person who contradicts her, she cannot tolerate it. Even when other two people are quarreling, she wants to beat the person who is at fault. She weeps a lot and keeps constantly thinking on the incident after the quarrel is over and wants to commit suicide. Then there is numbness and formicating feeling in occipital region and the headache begins. She dislikes crowds, as she feels nauseating and uncomfortable. She cannot stand frightful scenes. If the television is in loud sound, she gets irritated and turns off the set. If anybody increases the sound, it aggravates her chief complaint. She does not like sad songs they make her weep.

INTERPRETING PATIENT'S STORY: CASE I

Phase	Situation	Patient's Reactions	Interpretation
C H I L D H O O D [F A M I L Y]	When she was 3-4 years old mother did not come to pick her up from school. She started walking thinking that her home is near by but got lost. An autorikshaw driver picked her up and she stayed with him for 2 days, then he went to police to inform about her, meanwhile her parents also found her with the help of police.	She has bitter and painful memories of this incident. She felt very bad and started crying.	Insecurity
	She was born in a poor family. Parents could not afford even milk. Did not get milk after the age of 6 months. She was kept at her uncle's place from the age of 6yrs till she reached 12th standard, as her uncle didn't have a child and parents could not afford her upbringing.	She feels she was not given due care and attention at her uncle's place. It would have been much better if she had stayed with her parents.	Estrangement Loneliness

Phase	Situation	Patient's Reactions	Interpretation
ADOLESCENT	While staying at her uncle's place when she was in junior college, uncle used to keep face powder, hair oil etc. locked in a cupboard, didn't allow her to use cosmetics.	Felt very sad, wept a lot, got angry.	Unreasonable demands not met → Sadness
CELINZY (FAMILY)	When she was in 12th standard, her physics 'tutor' proposed her.	She said 'yes' and had an affair with him, wanted to marry him.	Infatuated
	Her uncle opposed her. Uncle thought she had a bad character, he spoke cheap things about her character.	She quarrelled with her uncle. She got very angry and beat up her uncle for making unjust remarks on her character. She hates him and has not seen her uncle's face since that day.	Anger / Hatred
ADULT (EARLY HOOD)	Her mother opposed her love marriage with physics tutor. Mother was of the opinion that her marriage would adversely affect her siblings future prospects.	She cancelled everything and didn't keep any contact with 'him' after that. She was mentally very upset.	Disappointment → Sadness

112

Phase	Situation	Patient's Reactions	Interpretation
EARLY BEFORE FAMILY	**Work** While working in a STD booth, she met her present husband. He belongs to a lower caste.	She got emotionally attached to him. She married him in June 2001.	Attachment → Infatuation
AFTER MARRIAGE UPTIL FIRST HOLY DAY	There was a strong opposition from parents from both sides, they did not keep contacts with them (patient and her husband). Parents of both sides never visit their home.	This makes her feel very sad and lonely. She had once thought that her mother in law would be like her mother and she will get care and attention which she didn't get earlier.	Frustration
ADULT HOOD	**During first pregnancy** There was no one to look after her. There was nobody whom she could tell her physical complaints and take help of, as she remained alone at home and nobody visited her. Now also, her husband goes out on duty and she is alone at home. Even	She was very depressed and used to weep a lot. She cannot concentrate on anything. She is constantly thinking, feeling sad	Depressed Forsaken →

Phase	Situation	Patient's Reactions	Interpretation
	while watching T.V. or taking lunch she thinks about everyone.	and lonely. Feels the deficiency of elders at home.	Brooding
	When she is alone in house	She feels fearful and bad thoughts come to her mind. She never wants to be alone and wants company.	Insecurity
C H I L D H O O D — F A M I L Y	**Childhood incident** While staying with parents when she was in 4th standard she was lying on a 'Khat' when her father came and pulled her arm and asked her to wash his clothes.	She has memories of that incident. She said she would do it later. She felt very irritated. She didn't keep any verbal communication with her father for next 6 months.	Hypersensitive → Anger
	Patient's description about her nature Whenever she is hurt	She weeps easily. She dislikes crowds as she feels nauseated and uncomfortable.	Hypersentive to Noise

Phase	Situation	Patient's Reactions	Interpretation
A D U L T H O O D	In crowds Frightful scenes	She cannot stand	**H Y P E R S E N S I T I V E**
	If the T.V. has loud sound	She gets irritated and turns off the T.V. set. It aggravates her chief complaint.	
	Sad songs	She does not like, they make her weep.	Sentimental
	Patient's description about her nature as a child	As a child, she could not accept no and must get whatever she asked for.	Demanding
		She must have anything she wanted immediately other wise used to cry a lot and create a scene. She was 'ziddi' type of child.	Adamant
C H I L D H O O D / **F A M I L Y**	**Adolescence** Father was a irritable person. She was the eldest amongst siblings	She always fought with her father for the rights of her siblings.	Demanding Quarrelsome
	After Marriage If her husband does not bring what she asked for	She gets angry and quarrels with him, weeps a lot. Does not accept the thing if it is brought later.	Demanding

115

Phase	Situation	Patient's Reactions	Interpretation
A D U L T H O O D	**Patient's description about her nature**		
A F T E R E P I S O D E	If somebody acts against her wishes and passes unjust remarks	She quarrels with that person.	Revengeful
Q U A R R E L S O M E	Whenever there is a dispute or altercation	She always takes the right side and stands by the truth as she cannot tolerate lies.	Adamant
	If anybody contradicts her	She starts trembling with anger and wants to beat the person who contradicts her. She cannot tolerate it.	Agitation → Anger
	Even when other two people are quarreling	She wants to beat the person who is at fault.	Quarrelsome
	After the quarrel is over	She weeps a lot and keeps constantly thinking on the incident and wants to commit suicide. Then there is numbness and formication feeling in occiput and the headache begins.	Brooding Vexation Frustration

The analysis of the patient's story emerge certain basic attributes, which are as follows:

Mental State:

- **Intellect :** Mediocre
- **Emotions:** Anger^{2+}
  Weepy
- **Behaviour :** Adamant
  Demanding^{2+}
  Brooding
- **Functioning :** Quarrelsome^{3+}
  Depressed
- **Expressions:**

Irritability	Disappointment
Agitation^{2+}	Brooding
Anger^{3+}	Sadness
Hatred	Weeping
Vexation	Frustration

Apparently, the case has some features resembling Magnesia, but the patient's mental state resembles more closely with Natrium muriaticum. Hence, it was selected as simillimum for the case.

ILLUSTRATIVE CASE II
(Interpreting patient's story)

Name: PT **Sex:** Female
Marriage: Unmarried **Religion:** Hindu
Occupation: Student, MA **Habits:** Vegetarian
Age: 29 years

Chief Complaints
- Joint pains
- Recurrent attacks of loose mucous stools

Patient's life story in her own words

I have a fair complexion and an average look. I am 5ft 4" tall and weigh 46kgs. I have a medium build. I love nature and have an attraction for all objects that are natural. I am friendly with plants and animals. I love them, caress them and talk to them. I love to be as close to them as possible. I love to do social work. I encourage and help those who need my help or who benefit from me such as poor people who are not aware of how to face challenges in life. It includes friends, family members as well as others in society. My own family does not accept and like me because I cannot be selfish and dirty natured like them. I believe in living with self respect, which is supreme to me. I do not talk to my father. He is a dirty man. I have broken off with him because he is a begot. His thoughts, speech, and actions are beastly. I do not like to see his face. I am lucky to have very good friends. I am quick to make friends. However, I am cautious while making them. I have very close relation with my cousins. The society loves me. I am spiritually inclined. I desire to inculcate spiritual values in me. I read books that impart such values and I have full faith in them. I have attended camps of 'Vipasana' and 'Art of living'; I have some inkling about the practice of reiki. I have attended Ramdeobaba's yoga camp also. I trust in the theory of awakening 'kundalini' in self. I trust saints and admire persons who have set ideals in their life and their teachings shall help me to achieve my ultimate goal. I do practice meditation. I fear God. I like to share the sorrows of others and try to help them out. I do not like to take credit for success. I do not like to be praised or acknowledged for efforts. My joy rests in their happiness. I do not have distinct memory of my childhood. However, I recall I was playful and enjoyed playing all games. I have two brothers, one elder and one younger. Currently my father is away from home. In childhood, I was very much afraid of my father and elder brother. There were too many restrictions for me at home. My brother used to beat me often. He was averse to noises and got angry whenever we youngsters made noise. I used to get irritated at him. I shuddered to go and ask his permission to do anything. My father used to go to the farm. Hence, my elder brother took over his responsibilities of managing us. Father was no different when he came home. He was very strict with all but especially with me. I being a girl, my mother was also very abusive and hit me. Because of this, I hated all of them. I felt, as a mother she should have been affectionate to her daughter more. However, that was not to be. Today, when I look back, I feel all this happened to me because of my ignorance. I developed a negative disposition towards my elders. Right from childhood, I felt nobody loved me. This feeling continues until today. I did not have any attachment for them in childhood; I do not have it even today. I always desired to go away from the oppressive environment at home. I lived in fear and felt much unsecured. I lived there under compulsion. My aunts were no different. One of my paternal aunts took me away to her house when I was studying in first standard on plea that she will improve my conduct. I still have distinct memory of the punishment she gave me. Apart from beatings, she tied me with a rope upside down, caused burns and scalds by lighting a matchstick or lamp against my skin, made me stand outside without a shred of cloth on me and so on. I developed a fear towards her and of that house. Even today, I do not want to recall those experiences and their unjust conduct. For them, it was a daily routine to punish me. I have terrible hatred towards my aunt and her husband. I grew in this atmosphere. I was an average student. I do not have anything to boast about my academic achievements. As I matured and started understanding the world around me, I realised many more things. It was one day after I graduated; my father did an act that was so detestable that I virtually quarrelled with him. It was one solitary occasion, I opened my mouth. I just could not accept his conduct. No one else in my position would have accepted him for that. I was mentally disturbed. Even then, my paternal aunts and their husbands spoke for him. They did not accept me. I wept continuously even as I was walking in or out of house. My friends and cousins came to my rescue. They consoled me and helped me get out of the terrible mental agony I suffered. I broke off completely with my father and aunts from that day. I have a hatred to hear their voices or for their sight. I started behaving like a crazy woman. All people around me felt that the only solution to my problem was to let me seek employment that will keep me away from home environment for the best part of the day. I accepted the proposal. However, it was not easy to put it through as my elder brother opposed it tooth and nail and on several occasions, I had to fight with him over the issue. My other brothers favoured it and sided me, especially the younger brother understood me more closely than the other did. I am the first female progeny to go for service in our family. To get a job I had to struggle and search for it myself. Nobody helped me. My own family members also did not help. My life has been full of struggle all the way. Even living in my own home has been a struggle. Education was a struggle; job was a struggle. Even marriage became a struggle. When any proposal for alliance came, she had to fight with rest of the family to exercise her choice. Even when I fell ill my elder brother, instead of being sympathetic abused me. Walking out of home for a job made me bold and infused greater confidence in myself. I never believed or did flattery of anybody. I earned and started attending college to do my post graduation in psychology. I did not ask for any money from home to pay my tuition fees. It hurt my ego to beg them for money. Home did not give me any needs or comfort. This is the tragedy of my life. I fell ill with joint pains 4 years ago. These gradually increased day by day and crippled my life. Medical treatment from different doctors did not help. I grew increasingly restive. It is under this stress that I worked out a change in my outlook. I developed my mind spiritually and changed my attitudes. I learnt to adjust with my family. I became sensitive to their feelings got closer to my mother. I became aware that she never had her husband's love and therefore has been conducting herself indifferently. I was very short tempered, angry and snobbish in younger days but much diluted now. When I started with my illness, it was a severe blow to my ego. I wept; thought it is the end road to me and loathed life. Thoughts of committing suicide often occurred to me. I cursed myself and god for choosing me for this punishment why was I singly punished? Why do I have to lead such a miserable life? At present, my thoughts have changed. My illness has given me a new life I thank my illness for that. It provided me greater contact with the world around me; newer and more lasting companions; a greater depth to know the real meaning of life. It offered me greater 'adhyatmic' power by which the people with evil thoughts distanced from me and those with spiritual leanings got closer. It is not that I have cut off from anybody; I still socialize with people whom I disliked. I discuss things with people I like. I do not get so much tensed now. Even if there is an occasion to feel tense, it gets over soon. There is a lot of difference in me today as compared to what I have been some years ago. My aspirations have changed. I aspire to take spiritual practices in life in the company of saints for whom I have an attraction from my childhood. I aspire to work for upliftment of poor and do social work. I have grown in wisdom and have succeeded in shaping my aspirations that I had at 14 or 15 years of age to their logical end. I am deeply aware that I need to make many efforts ahead of me to attain what I have set for me. It is therefore, I need to recover faster from my illness so that the time does not run out for me. Marriage has never attracted me in either the past or now. I do not regard it as an essential condition of life. I yearn to spend rest of my life in an ashram amongst people and serve them.

Physician's notes during Case taking

She has been an average student all through. Her education suffered initially because her paternal aunt took her away for improving her conduct when she was six years old and studying in first standard. She lost a year of schooling. The experiences she had there and the subsequent treatment by her parents and siblings was responsible for average performance in school. Somehow, she did her matriculation and 12th standard passing with higher second-class marks. She graduated in 1998 and then until 2001 she did a job. She had to resign from her job not only because of her mother's illness but also marriage proposals began coming. She has joined a correspondence course in psychotherapy and counselling. She has appeared in MPSC examination in December last year, the results of which is awaited. Now she aspires to take a job through UPSC after she gets well.

Her mother is meek. Never retorts. Her in-laws treated her badly, she tolerated it quietly.

Her father was a womanizer. He had affair with a nurse after birth of his child and he married her. 6 years ago when he was admitted for fever in a local hospital, she learnt about his relations with another woman. She was shocked. She was aghast that even after his age of 50 years he was so lascivious. She wept and regarded him as a beast. That was the incident she had mentioned in the write up that made her fight with him. She told him she felt ashamed to call him her father. He is not worthy of being one. Her objection had no effect on him. He refused to relent for his actions. Instead, he argued he did no wrong. Her aunts and their husbands supported him and said there was nothing wrong in his conduct. She narrated the event to her cousins. They were the only sympathizers with her. These events made her cut off all relations with her father and stop communicating with him.

At her age of 6 years when she stayed with paternal aunt, she did manual work and took care of younger children. She received no love but only punishment even though she worked all day. She felt her aunt was using her. She hated them. However, she was equally afraid of her and could not open her mouth, she kept crying silently. Looking back, she regards her aunt and uncle as persons belonging to lower strata and they derived a lot of pleasure doing unjust things for creating quarrels. She has stopped visiting them since 6 years.

The sense she had of her childhood experiences was that she was forsaken.

She admitted that being a woman she has to marry but that will be only to fulfill social obligation.

She looked tense and depressed. Hence, she decided to work. She took a job as office administrator and computer operator for 2 years. However, she had to resign due to her mother's illness at first and then because of her own illness.

She firmly beliefs that her twelve day stint in a meditation camp helped her resolve all her problems.

INTERPRETING PATIENT'S STORY: CASE II

Phase	Situation	Patient's Reactions	Interpretation
C H I L D H O O D / F A M I L Y	About elder brother and father	Afraid of father and elder brother.	Fear
	Brother got angry when youngsters made noises.	Used to get irritated at him.	Anger
	Brother used to beat her often.	(I shuddered to go and ask his permission to do anything).	Fear
	Father was very strict especially with her.	Felt that as a mother she should have been affectionate to her daughter.	Sense of Rejection
	Mother was bad tongued, abusive and hit her	Had hatred for all of them.	Anger → Hatred
		Developed negative disposition towards elders. Felt nobody loved her, this feeling continues until today.	Sense of Rejection
		Didn't have any attachement for them in childhood (I don't have it even today).	Estrangment

Phase	Situation	Patient's Reactions	Interpretation
CHILDHOOD FAMILY		Desired to go away from oppressive environment at home. I lived in fear and felt very insecure.	Insecurity
	About her childhood experiences	She has a sense of being forsaken.	Forsaken
	Aunt took her away on plea of improving her conduct. Punished her.	She developed fear towards her and that house. Even today does not want to recall those experiences and unjust conduct.	Insecurity
EARLY ADULT FAMILY LIFYHOOD		She has terrible hatred towards her aunt and her husband.	Hostility
	Event after her graduation, father did an act that was detestable	Quarrelled with him, was mentally disturbed, wept continuously.	Indignation → Anger →
		Broke of completely with father and aunts from that day. (I have hatred to hear their voices or sight).	Sadness Hatred

125

Phase	Situation	Patient's Reactions	Interpretation
ADULTHOOD / FAMILY	When she learnt about fathers relations with another women	She was shocked and aghast that even after his age of 50 years he was so lascivious, felt ashamed to call him her father. She wept, regarded him as beast, this was the incident that made her fight with him.	Mortification → Disgust → Anger
	People around her felt that letting her seek employment was the only solution to her problem, she also accepted it. Elder brother opposed it.	She faught with him over the issue on several occasion.	Adamant
	When any proposal for alliance came	She had to fight with rest of the family to exercise her choice	Demanding Selfwilled
	To do post graduation	She earned and started attending college, didn't ask for any money from home to pay her tuition fees. It hurts her ego to beg them for money.	Self respect ← Wants to be independent

Phase	Situation	Patient's Reactions	Interpretation
A D U L T F A M I L Y H O O D	When she fell ill (her thoughts about herself and her illness)	It was a severe blow to her ego. She wept, thought it is the end and loathed life, thoughts of committing suicide often occurred to her (I cursed myself and god for choosing me for the punishment, why am I singly punished? Why do I have to lead such a miserable life).	Depression → Frustration
A D U L T H O O D	Her thoughts about herself and her illness	Her illness has given her a new life and she thanks her illness for that, it has provided her with greater contact with world around her and new and more lasting companions, a greater depth to know real meaning of life. It has offered her greater 'adhyatmic' power.	Delusion
	About her 12 day stint in meditation camp.	She firmly believes it has helped her resolve all her problems.	

Phase	Situation	Patient's Reactions	Interpretation
ADULTHOOD WORK		She says her aspirations have changed, she aspires to take spiritual practices in life in company of saints for whom she has attraction from childhood. Aspires to work for upliftment of poor and do social work.	Delusion
		She has grown in wisdom and has succeeded in shaping her aspirations she had at 14 -15 years of age to their logical end.	Delusion
EARLY ADULTHOOD	WORK School	Lost years of schooling because aunt took her away for improving her conduct.	
	Matric and 12th	Average performance higher second class marks.	Mediocre
	1998 - 2001 Graduated, did a job.	Had to resign her job due to mother's illness and marriage proposals began coming.	

Phase	Situation	Patient's Reactions	Interpretation
A D U L T H O O D	Worked as office administrator and computer operator	She had to resign due to her mother's illness at first and then because of her own illness for 2 years.	Changeability. →
		She joined correspondence course in psychotherapy and counselling. Appeared in MPSC exam in Dec. last year. Aspires to take a job through UPSC after she gets well.	Contradiction → Confusion
	Her views about marriage.	It has never attracted her in the past or now. She says she does not regard it as an essential condition of life.	Pretence ←
		She says, she yearns to spend the rest of her life in an ashram amongst people and serve them.	Frustration Confusion

The analysis of the patient's story emerge certain basic attributes, which are as follows:

Mental State:

- **Intellect:** Mediocre
  Delusion^{2+}
  Confusion^{2+}
  Ego^{+}
- **Emotions:** Need – Demand Conflict
  Sense of Rejection
  Anger^{2+}
- **Behaviour:** Demanding^{2-}
  Contradictory
- **Functioning:** Changeable
  Repressive
- **Expressions:**

Irritability	Brooding
Anger^{3+}	Sadness
Hatred	Weeping
Vexation	Frustration^{3+}
Disappointment	

Patient's mental state resembles more closely with Magnesia group. Hence remedy from Magnesia group would have to be selected as simillimum for the case.

A CASE FOR WORKING
(Interpretation of patient's mind from patient's life story)

Directions for working
- Read the following case (History given by the patient and the physician's notes) carefully
- Examine the reactions of the patient to situations faced during different phases in his life in all areas
- Interpret the reactions with relation to the situations to arrive at the basic emotions causing them. Evolve the traits and expressions with strict relation to time to elicit the psychodynamics in this case. Match it with the similar psychodynamics of the drug study that has been evolved and documented to arrive at the group to which the patient belongs.

Purpose
When the above study is seen in conjunction with the physical and pathological generals of the case and differentiated with the aid of characteristic particulars, the simillimum for the case in its totality is perceived.

Name: Dr J. D.   **Age:** 51 years

Sex: Male   **Occupation:** General Surgeon

Habit: Vegetarian   **Marriage:** Yes

Chief Complaint
- Chronic complaint of recurrent tonsillo-pharyngitis
- Bowel irregularities
- Acidity

He is fair and moderate in built. His height is 5'7"and weight is 65 kgs.

Details of Case taking

He was from a lower middle class family. He had just 1-2 dresses and had to pull on with them. He was little hesitant, subdued and overcautious due to that. He felt others had four dresses and why he had just one or two. He did share his things with his brother and friends but there wasn't much to share. Whenever he had a fight with his brother he took care that his brother should not be hurt. He was a responsible child yet on occasions unnecessarily reacted against his father and mother. His childhood needs were not fulfilled and he was disappointed over that. Once he wanted a school bag and didn't get it, he felt sad and couldn't do anything. In class, when a question was asked he was hesitant and since he didn't have command over english even if he knew the answer couldn't express. He got 60% at school, took efforts to improve english and got 74% at inter examination. He was impressionable, carried away with friend's talks and told his personal feelings unhesitatingly to them. He put his trust on them yet they cheated him. A childhood friend as well as his classmate was his companion for thirty years. He shared with him whatever the minimum he had. Now whenever his friend visits he feels he comes with some interest and in the past too had some motive to help him. He was in love with a girl from other caste. He could not marry her. Now feels if he married her his career would have been spoiled and he would have lost track. He has got a very good wife and thanks god for that. During professional graduation and post graduation exams, he always got anxious and on few occasions took sedatives. His performance was good all through. He improved his english. He passed with good marks throughout. He has cordial relations with his daughter and wife and greatly attached with them. If things in house are not kept properly, he reacts sharply, does loose temper and is harsh too sometimes. He cannot control his anger. He stays in an apartment and when people coming to the neighbours; park their vehicles at wrong places obstructing his way or on his parking place he will object to it and will point it strongly and sternly, he tends to loose temper but tries to control it. When this repeatedly happened he parked his scooter in a manner that it will obstruct the moving of the wrongly parked vehicles. The angry neighbours called him and everybody felt a brawl was sure. He put his point strongly and clearly that in spite of his repeated telling they didn't correct themselves. Removed his scooter and while going back invited them for a cup of coffee. He tries to cool down things after acrimony. Doesn't let go things out of control even if looses temper. He is fine in his work. The operations performed by him leave least scars. Wherever he worked, was appreciated by seniors as well as juniors. His submission to work is total. Says, he is abnormally sincere, perfect, clear and accountable to patients. He used to cancel surgeries on operation tables if he felt it was not really needed and he would go by his own assessment. In a surgical case no surgeon was ready to operate but he went ahead with an impossible and unique surgery and he was successful which was a miracle, was confident due to submission to god. His boss treated all his subordinates badly and finally he decided to quit. The boss came to know and asked 'you are thinking to quit I have learned'. He replied sharply 'No Sir, I have already left'. He and others tried to pursue and convince him not to leave but there was no looking back, he left and didn't bother about the effects. About his past boss says, he was an egoist, you have to treat subordinate well, unnecessary bossism doesn't help. Small happenings disturb him he can't sleep thinks about them, does well and still can't sleep. He honestly worked everywhere, never compromised with his principles, says money can never buy him. His practice doesn't match his skills about which he blames destiny. Perhaps a flourishing practice is not destined for him. He was having a small house at a 'taluka' place but due to his daughter's future and property dispute he moved from there and started new clinic in a city. He was hesitant but prepared for every eventuality; he says 'if you are intellectual type you have more subconscious anxiety.' Before surgery, he has anxiety of evacuation. Has anxiety even if his wife has some assignment. During his presentation at a national conference, he was hesitant but went on dais and presented confidently. People liked him, he says he is always hesitant to come on stage and perform. He doesn't hesitate to meet general physicians to explain his approach to surgical cases (mostly conservative) and request them to send patients, but doesn't indulge in cut or percentage practice. His brother has managed to transfer his entire father's property to himself. He has filed a legal suit, says no grudge about him nor wants to do bad to him but since he is basically a rebellion, does reprimand to scare him and tell him if you can shout aloud I can shout ten times more. He is more attached to his mother and he has been mother's pet child. No soreness about father, does meet both of them regularly. He has been cordial with relatives but because of their rude behaviour he too retaliated by speaking sharply. He says he will retaliate but with lawful means. He used to react sharply in the past. He will dominate those who are jealous, couldn't tolerate injustice and unjust behaviour. He is sensitive and little things disturb him. He is a ruthless spender. He used to criticise very badly but it was ironical and witty not sarcastic, says there is a difference. He is quick to point faults. He always reacted sharply hence his relations spoiled. His honesty and integrity are his greatest assets and not acceptable. People feel it is modified and false. He is yet to find a person who is nearby to his attitude about honesty. People misinterpret him most of the times. He is a fighter, can't tolerate injustice. A programme in his area created a lot of noise pollution for 8 days. He gathered people, lodged a police complaint, and has been chasing the issue till now. A man in a shopping mall was counting notes by applying saliva. He immediately complained the manager and put a note in the complain box. On the helmet issue he says how inconvenient it is for old people, children and patients (with spondylitis). He does not wear a helmet and is waiting for someone to catch him. He carries a rebellion attitude for injustice. He gets irritated from bottom of heart. Now carries a spiritual attitude. On Palestine- Israel issue and terrorism in India he says we must learn from Israel, so many people have died in our country and still we haven't retaliated.

He presently reads spiritual books, organizes spiritual programmes, loves helping needy people and advices earnestly. Attainment of salvation is the only aim. Now analyses everything in spiritual light.

His behaviour with the physician:

He appeared anxious about trivial complaints, frequently calls up physician and worried about complications. He says physician must be aware about each and every smallest change, hence calls up. He always greets very warmly, follows formalities like 'thank you so much', 'sorry to trouble you', 'bye' etc, talks excessively and fast.

The various interpretations are as follows:

- Ambitious
- Desire to rise up
- Sincere
- Fastidious
- Egoist
- Attachment^{2+}
- Sensitive
- Disappointment
- Vexation
- Brooding
- Irritable
- Snappy
- Censorious
- Hatred
- Jealous
- Agitation Anxiety
- Anticipatory Anxiety
- Fear
- Insecurity
- Discouraged
- Philosophical
- Faith in God and Guru

Mental State
- Intellect: Above average
- Motivated
- Conscientious
- Emotion: Anger³⁺
- Sentimental³⁺
- Anxiety³⁺
- Behaviour: Excitable
- Functioning: Uncompromising
- Rebellious

CHAPTER 6

Clinical Diagnosis

- ❖ Value of Diagnosis 140
- ❖ Steps in Diagnosis 144

CHAPTER 6

CLINICAL DIAGNOSIS

The term diagnosis consists of 'dia' which means through and 'gnosis' which means recognizing. Thus diagnosis means the art of recognizing the disease the patient is suffering from, or it simply means labeling of a 'disease.' Famous German philosopher Immanuel Kant (1724-1804) once remarked sullenly, "Physicians think they do a lot for a patient when they give his disease a name." Similarly Hahnemann too criticized mere labeling of diseases and emphasized the study of individual suffering from disease. He has repeatedly stressed on the symptomatological basis of homeopathic prescription in his Organon of Medicine. Thus since the time of Hahnemann it got firmly implanted in the minds of majority of homeopaths that the choice of remedy is decided upon by the symptoms outside the diagnostic sphere. As a result we still find a section of homeopaths and lay practitioners totally neglecting the nomenclature of the disease and the pathology involved with it. But a homeopath cannot afford to part with diagnosis. Homeopath like any other physician is a diagnostician too. The difference is that his concept of diagnosis is wide ranging. He has to diagnose multiple phenomenons.

Components are:
- Pathological diagnosis.
- Remedial diagnosis.
- Miasmatic diagnosis.

First comes the disease diagnosis, which relates to the pathology, then the remedial diagnosis and last but not the least miasmatic diagnosis which deals with 'Hahnemannian pathology' i.e. the miasms.

VALUE OF DIAGNOSIS

DIAGNOSIS HELPS THE HOMEOPATH IN :

- Identity of disease.
- Selection of cases.
- Disease curable or incurable.
- Predicting the time required for recovery and prognosis.
- Prevention.
- Advising diet and regimen.
- Taking prophylactic measures.
- Knowing the seat of disease.
- Staged disease.
- Issuing sickness certificates.
- Proving that homeopathy is scientific.
- Maintaining statistics.
- Differentiating disease symptoms from patient's symptoms.
- Remedy selection.
- Indicating the contraindications for certain type of remedies.
- Potency selection.
- Recognizing dominant miasm in the case.
- Second prescription.

Although the art of labeling diseases has always been subservient to the art of individualizing and selecting the simillimum, still a homeopath should not neglect it. Diagnosis has multitude of advantages in store for a physician who does it correctly. Diagnosis establishes identity of the disease, which is the first step towards establishing the individuality of the patient, which the homeopath wants to accomplish. Patients in general recognize the diseases by their names; therefore, the patient who seeks our consultation wants to know the name of the disease he is suffering from. He also wants to know whether his disease is curable or not? What things he should avoid indulgence in for a faster recovery from his ailment? The approximate period required to relieve him completely. A physician is expected to know answers to all these questions after he has thoroughly examined the patient both physically as well as through clinical interview. The answers to all these questions lie in physician's ability to diagnose the diseases accurately.

Physician should be precise in diagnosis. Kent has also stressed on the importance of correct diagnosis in homeopathic practice in his lectures on homeopathic philosophy. He says that, *"Diagnosis is something that a physician cannot be foolish about. He cannot afford to be a blunderer; he cannot afford to go around calling scarlet fever measles and measles scarlet fever. He must know enough about the general nature of diseases that after the prescription has been made and the patient settled as to that, and the mother wants to know what is the matter with the child, to tell her, for in that instance, she has a perfect right to know that is a case where the family must be protected. Where outsiders must be protected, the physician must decide whether it is proper for the child to go to school or whether it is not proper."* Kent also gives some practical implications of diagnosis. He states that name of the disease is important because, board of health expects a doctor to mention the particular disease patient died from. Recognizing disease is necessary when a physician comes in contact with the world.

Several other advantages lie inherent in diagnosing the disease, apart from those mentioned by Kent. Diagnosis considerably augments physician's potential to handle various cases skillfully. A true homeopath never tries to play god and never makes false claims; he selects his cases before treating them. He knows what is curable, what needs palliation, and what falls out of the range of operation of homeopathy. Only a physician who is fully conversant with diagnostic and pathological aspect of disease is able to do this. Selection of cases is most important to avoid pitfalls in practice. Diagnosis helps the physician to select his cases; it also makes him capable of advising the patient with regards to prognosis of the disease, the restrictions regarding the type of diet and mode of living. Therefore, it helps the physician in removing the obstacles in the way of recovery.

Diagnosis also serves as a 'filter' of symptoms; with diagnosis one is able to discard common symptoms keeping only uncommon symptoms, which are of prime importance in remedial diagnosis. It also helps the physician in guiding the community as regards to prophylactic measures in case of epidemics. It also plays a vital role in indicating the do's and don'ts and contraindications as regards to choice of potency, for example, in cases of advanced pathological changes, deep acting drugs in high potency and frequent repetition are strictly contraindicated. A physician who neglects this might land into serious trouble as improper selection of remedy and potency in case of advanced pathological changes can lead to disastrous results.

At times the symptoms which seem to be very peculiar, might be the result of some mechanical causes, as in case of pressure symptoms due to tumors etc. and in such cases diagnosis of the ailment will make it clear that these symptoms are not worth considering for homeopathic prescribing. Diagnosis is also necessary for knowing the exact seat of the disease. Although location is of secondary importance in homeopathic prescribing it may guide at times in indicating a remedy, as certain remedies have a special affinity for certain organs or locations and thus are frequently indicated in disease conditions affecting those organs. Similarly, certain medicines come into consideration in certain stage of the disease, for example, Pulsatilla is never indicated in first stage of coryza. Disease diagnosis also helps the physician in proper interpretation of the results after first prescription is made by making him able to differentiate the symptoms due to natural progress of the disease from those symptoms, which are due to action of the prescribed remedy. Thus, indicating as to the correctness of the prescription.

Diagnosis may prove helpful in repertorizing cases with advanced pathology, as the characteristics are deficient in such cases due to the gross pathological changes. Pathological generals are used to repertorize such cases using Boger-Boenninghausen's repertory. Apart form those mentioned earlier diagnosis serves many miscellaneous purposes such as maintaining statistics of type of diseases successfully treated with homeopathy, for research work and case presentation. It is necessary to mention the name of the disease while issuing sickness and death certificates; nomenclature of disease comes handy here too.

A physician should not hesitate to advise the patient to undergo laboratory investigations and pathological tests prior to treatment and after the complaints are ameliorated, whenever necessary. Pathological tests carried out before beginning the homeopathic treatment and after the patient reports disappearance of symptoms during the course of homeopathic treatment serve as a means of establishing the scientific approach and efficiency of the treating physician and homeopathy as well. We can conclude that nomenclature of disease has multiple advantages for a homeopath and therefore in spite of the fact that the study of the individual is more important for a homeopath, still he can't neglect diagnosis which is complementary to the study of the individual.

STEPS IN DIAGNOSIS

A methodical approach, involving step-by-step evaluation of the patient from diagnostic point of view is necessary for accuracy in diagnosis. The main steps in disease diagnosis accepted by all the medical sciences are as follows:

1. Interpretation of clinical features.
2. Physical examination.
3. Investigations.
4. Differential diagnosis.

1. INTERPRETATION OF CLINICAL FEATURES

Its components include:
- Disordered function and structure.
- Pathology.
- Diagnosis.
- Seat of disease.
- Modalities of disease.
- Sensations.
- Etiological factors.

The first step in labeling the disease process is the interpretation of clinical features in terms of disordered function and structure and in terms of pathology if the latter can be demonstrated. Every disease has its own characteristic clinical features like the remedies in materia medica which have their individual characteristics. Many a times these characteristics of the disease can directly point to the diagnosis if properly interpreted

Clinical Diagnosis

with reference to organ or system involved. Rational interpretation of clinical features demands knowledge of clinical medicine (which Hahnemann described as knowledge of disease in the third paragraph of Organon.). The complaints of the patient can belong to the organ or system affected due to disease or sometimes the complaints belong to other systems or organs away from the system which is affected. All this must be kept in mind for accurate interpretation of symptoms or clinical features. For example, pain during micturition and changes in colour of urine point to the urinary system. Whereas sometimes the patient comes with drowsiness, persistent nausea and vomiting which may be due to uraemia but here the symptoms belong to other systems. The modalities also need to be taken into consideration during interpretation of clinical features. Like the remedies which have characteristic modalities the diseases too have modalities which characterize them.

Some examples are as follows:

- A pain in center of chest which is aggravated after exertion or climbing stairs is almost certainly due to ischaemia of the heart (angina). A similar pain which is aggravated after eating is probably esophageal.
- Pain in abdomen which is promptly relieved by eating is characteristic of duodenal ulcer.
- Headache of migraine is made worse by jolting or movement and bright light, whereas a psychogenic headache is likely to be increased by emotional stress or mental fatigue. Lying down position makes the headache of sinusitis more intense but subsequently it subsides.

The location or site of the complaint also gives idea about the organ or system involved and contributes to diagnostic evaluation. For example, pain in upper abdomen suggests diseases of gastric or duodenal origin. Pancreatitis and cholecystitis also come into picture. Pain in right iliac fossa is commonly due to appendicitis. Lower abdominal pain points to diseases of bladder and prostate and in females it might be due to diseases of female pelvic organs. Sometimes the site of the disease is a sure indication of the diagnosis. For example, pain in single joint is probably due to infection, hemarthrosis and psoriatic arthritis. In rheumatoid arthritis, there is symmetrical involvement of joints, while in osteoarthritis or gout the joint involvement is asymmetrical.

The sensations cannot be explained on the basis of pathology for remedy selection. The physicians should takes a special note of 'sensation as if' and peculiar, strange and queer type of sensations. He also has to take into consideration the type of sensations from diagnostic point of view. Sensations sometimes assume an important place in disease diagnosis.

Here are some examples:

- A spasmodic type of pain in abdomen suggests a renal background or it might be due to abdominal infection and in females due to uterine contractions as in dysmenorrhea.
- In peritonitis the pain does not wax and wane but is of steady type.
- Burning pain in middle of chest is often due to hyperacidity and is of gastric origin, whereas a sensation of constriction or a band-like sensation in the middle of chest suggests cardiac disease or angina.
- The cardiac pains usually extend to left arm and may be associated with tingling sensation and numbness of fingers.

Thus, we can conclude that the location, sensations and the modalities play a vital role in remedial diagnosis as well as the disease diagnosis.

The past history and family history may hint at the probable etiological factor, therefore needs to be looked into along with clinical features.

2. PHYSICAL EXAMINATION

Homeopathic practitioners in general seem to be ignorant about the physical examination, although Hahnemann and other stalwarts never said that a homeopath should not do physical examination. It is as important for a homeopath as it is for an allopath. Physical examination provides important information regarding functioning of organs and structural changes if any. Physician uses his senses of vision, touch, hearing and smell in order to compare patient's structure with the normal and to assess his body function. A physical examination from head to toe may not be necessary in every patient that comes to us. The nature of examination should be decided considering the type of complaints.

It is a common misconception that physical examination begins when the patient is laid on the examination table. But it begins from observing the patient. Apart from routine examination which involves measurement of pulse, B.P. auscultation and percussion, the observation of the patient is also necessary. His appearance, postures way of standing and sitting, etc. should be taken note of. This is also an integral part of physical examination and may point to disease as well as the remedy. The characteristic facies of various diseases like hypothyroidism, thyrotoxicosis, acromegaly, third and seventh cranial nerve palsy, etc. are examples of observation of patient's face leading to diagnosis. The parotid swellings are obvious on inspection of face in patient of mumps. The examination of skin also at times indicates the probable disease, as in hemolytic jaundice the skin looks yellow. The dry and inelastic skin of dehydration is also well known. Cyanosis suggests imperfect oxygenation of blood. Presence of bony nodules in finger joints is typical of osteoarthritis. Many such examples can be given to highlight the importance of observation in diagnosis.

Procedures like auscultation and percussion give information about the bowel sounds, heart sounds, and murmurs and thus aid in diagnosis. Even a homeopath must learn these methods in his internship period, as it would prove beneficial in diagnostic evaluation of patients in his private practice. In severely ill patients a good physical examination reveals to the physician, whether the patient can be treated homeopathically or he needs immediate hospital care.

3. INVESTIGATIONS

The investigative procedures have progressed a great deal in recent years. There is growing tendency to depend upon investigations for diagnosis amongst allopaths for which they are criticized. The cost of investigations has increased by leaps and bounds. An average patient cannot afford costly tests; therefore, he might come to a homeopath expecting him to be in a position to treat without laboratory investigations and tests. However, a homeopath also sometimes requires certain pathological tests in order to assess the patient's condition and to diagnose the disease. A homeopath has to be rational in his approach towards advising investigations to be done. He must know what investigations and their necessity to request in given circumstances. The discomfort and possible risk to the patient of an investigation also needs to be looked into. The approximate cost in time and money must be kept in mind before asking the patient to do a certain test.

The result of any laboratory investigation is only one part of the information required to make diagnosis. It may have as much or as little significance as any other physical finding.

The type of investigations has to be decided from facts obtained through case taking and physical examination. The tests should not be repeated frequently without good logical reason. While referring the patient to pathologist or radiologist, the complaints of the patient and probable diagnosis should be stated in the reference letter. Any therapy or drugs that might influence biochemical investigations should also be recorded. It is advisable to write patient's full name in the reference letter so that the confusion arising out of similar family names is avoided.

Interpretation of any investigation depends on the relevance of the test to probable diagnosis. It is also largely dependent upon the physician's knowledge of pathology, biochemistry and physiology. Pathology today is a specialized subject, new investigative procedures are emerging everyday. A homeopath is expected to be familiar with them although he cannot be expected to have a detailed knowledge of each.

4. DIFFERENTIAL DIAGNOSIS

The most important step in diagnosis is the differentiation between similar clinical pictures. It is somewhat like the one done for remedy selection where the characteristics of remedies are differentiated. Differentiation of similar clinical pictures is possible only when the physician knows the details of each disease in question that resembles the patient's diagnostic symptoms. A careful student of clinical medicine always emerges a winner, if he is able to spot the hallmarks of the disease. Diseases express themselves through typical symptom presentation and clinical findings characterize them.

Few examples are :

- Absence of koplik's spots rules out measles. Typical distribution of eruptions and the 'teardrop' vesicles typical of chickenpox differentiate it from other eruptive diseases.
- Fever of malaria can be differentiated from typhoid by its pattern. Malarial fever declines and touches normal where as the typhoid fever shows remissions but never touches normal and also there is a stepladder rise in fever.

CHAPTER 7

Integrated Approach to Case Processing

- ❖ Concept of Analysis 155
- ❖ Types of Symptoms 157
- ❖ Generals 164
- ❖ Particulars 169
- ❖ Concept of Evaluation in Practice 170
- ❖ Synthesis of Case 172

CHAPTER 7

INTEGRATED APPROACH TO CASE PROCESSING

Once the diagnosis is done, it brings the physician to another important element in homeopathic practice and that is study of the individual or in other words case processing.

Following is a diagrammatic representation of homeopathic case processing:

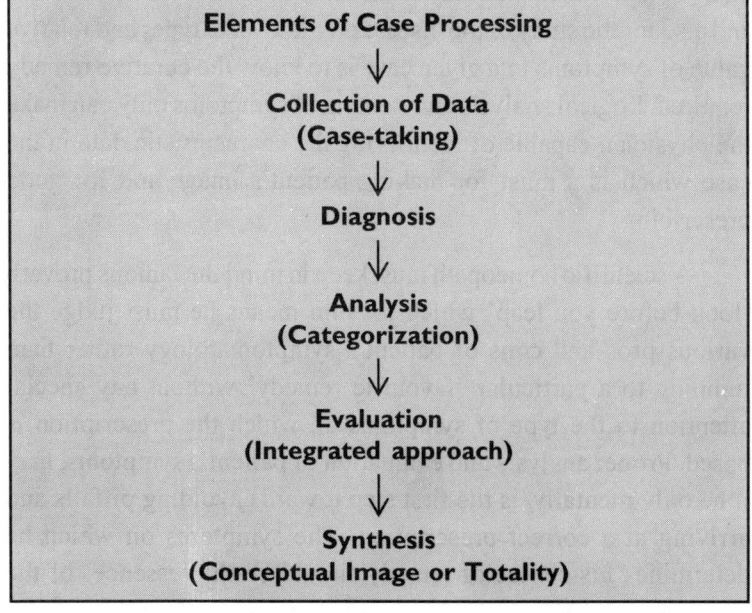

Study of the patient in systematic manner is must in order to erect totality in full accord with the principles of homeopathy, therefore the most important part of homeopathic practice is scrutinizing and processing the information obtained during case taking. It involves three main procedures: Analysis, Evaluation and Synthesis. All these procedures are centered around understanding the symptomatology of the case and therefore, after a thorough case taking and diagnosis is done, the third step towards discovery of simillimum is distillation of patient's symptomatology, which involves analysis and evaluation. Proper analysis and evaluation is the base for curative prescription.

Homeopathy considers symptoms as the language of the disease. A qualitative appreciation of the various symptoms is a must if the physician wishes to understand this language. Physician can understand the language of symptoms only after they are graded logically; without it physician is sure to get lost in the unfiltered maze of symptoms. Evaluation of symptoms is necessary for the study of individual, the study of the remedies in our materia medica and also for the study of the diseases. To know the types and relative value of symptoms in a given case is to know the curative remedy required. Logical analysis and ranking of symptoms only can make the physician capable of identifying the characteristic data in the case which is a must for making patient's image and for good prescribing.

A scientific homeopath must keep in mind the famous proverb 'look before you leap' which for him means he must judge the various pros and cons of patient's symptomatology rather than jumping to a particular 'favourite remedy' without any special attention to the type of symptoms on which the prescription is based. Proper analysis and evaluation of patient's symptoms, may it be only mentally, is the first step towards avoiding pitfalls and arriving at a correct prescription. The symptoms on which he determines his choice of remedy should be the 'essence' of the case in hand and the process carried out to get this essence is called as the analysis and evaluation of symptoms. Knowledge of pathology, medicine and knowledge of practical implications of the philosophical concepts advanced by various stalwarts is a prerequisite and contributory to proper case analysis and evaluation. Key to successful homeopathic practice lies in physician's ability to discriminate the symptoms of the individual from the symptoms of the disease.

CONCEPT OF ANALYSIS

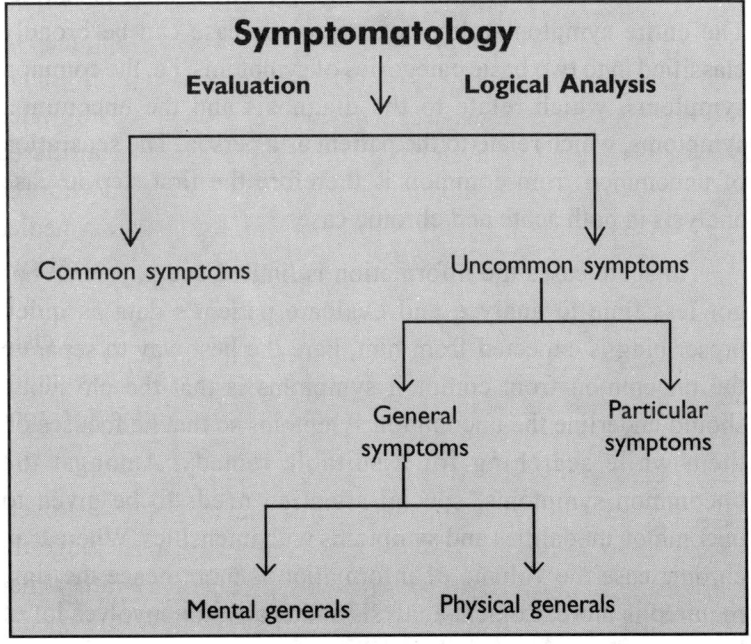

Aim of the physician in case analysis and evaluation is reaching the 'characteristic data' all-important for him. In the characteristic data lies the scientific solution of case. Qualitative appreciation of patient's symptomatology is the only route to simillimum for a homeopath. Analysis of symptoms is the first step towards this purpose. Case-analysis can be defined as the process of splitting the patient's symptomatology to identify and categorize symptoms into various classes, or in other words it is identification of elements of the case in hand. Analysis makes the task of evaluation easier. Analysis involves division and subdivision of attributes or symptoms of the case and also regrouping of symptoms. It is the assortment of the data to make various parts of the data recognizable, so that later these parts can be fitted together to make a meaningful whole. The meaningful whole is the totality. But there is likelihood of conceptual errors while analyzing a case due to inability to identify symptoms. The question therefore follows, how to analyze a case properly? The answer is simple. The entire symptomatology of any given case can be broadly classified in to two basic categories of symptoms, i.e. the common symptoms, which relate to the diagnosis and the uncommon symptoms, which relate to the patient as a person. The separation of uncommon from common is therefore the first step in case analysis in both acute and chronic cases.

In acute cases the information is limited and physician has got less time to analyze and evaluate patient's data as quick prescribing is expected from him, here the best way to separate the uncommon from common symptoms is that the physician should underline the uncommon symptoms so that he focuses on them while searching for a suitable remedy. Amongst the uncommon symptoms, special attention needs to be given to uncommon modalities and symptoms with intensities. Whereas in chronic case the volume of information is more hence the time required is more. Logical analysis and evaluation involves lot of brainstorming and especially in chronic cases requires considerable patience on part of the physician before putting a stamp on particular remedy. For a beginner who requires more time to do it the best way is by administering placebo after case taking and asking the patient to report after 2-3 days whenever possible so that the physician gets time to analyze the case properly. In chronic cases he should do it in writing which makes the job less confusing and easier. Physician should make two columns with headings—Common symptoms and Uncommon symptoms, and then the relevant symptoms should be put under these headings. Next is separating from the uncommon symptoms the generals and particulars. The generals should be further separated into mental and physical generals. This transfer of symptoms into various compartments would make the symptomatology of the case more intelligible to the physician. Correct analysis makes the job of evaluation easy. Such detailed analysis requires hard work and concentration. A new practitioner should make it a habit to do such analysis preferably in writing. It often proves beneficial in the long run as repeated analysis of cases improves ones understanding of symptomatology and matters related to it such as repertorization, totality perceiving and drug selection.

It is important to keep in mind that if the common symptom is having intensity it becomes uncommon. If a common symptom appears periodically it cannot be considered as common and becomes characteristic. Two common symptoms alternating with each other become uncommon. If a physician fails to pay attention to these points and is mechanical in his approach then he is likely to make mistakes in analyzing the case. Analysis is the first step towards making a conceptual image of the patient. After analysis of symptoms as described earlier physician has a list of uncommon symptoms with relevant classification of symptoms of the case.

TYPES OF SYMPTOMS

Proper analysis requires a physician to be well conversant with the classification of symptoms. Theoretical insight into the categorization of symptoms makes the job of analysis and synthesis easy and quick. Homeopaths since Hahnemann's time have used varied nomenclature for describing various types of symptoms. Due to the vastness of phraseology used by them the study of symptomatology becomes difficult. According to Dr. Jugal Kishor, there are at least 50 types of symptoms described in homeopathic literature till now. The same symptom is described by four different names by four different stalwarts. This is very perplexing for a beginner. An all-embracing, comprehensive nomenclature and classification is therefore very necessary in practice if one is to master the science of symptomatology, which is a first step towards identifying patient's image and differentiating various images in materia medica. As already stated, all the symptoms which a physician comes across in studying a patient or a remedy in homeopathic materia medica can be classified into two broad categories:

1. Common symptoms.
2. Uncommon or Characteristic symptoms.

1. COMMON SYMPTOMS

The symptoms of the disease or the symptoms with pathological basis are called common symptoms. Similarly the symptoms which are produced by large number of remedies are also called as common symptoms. They are the symptoms of 'Allopathic type,' for example dyspnea is a common symptom in majority of respiratory diseases. Although they play important role in diagnosis, but are not useful for individualization. Common symptoms are known by various other names such as:

(a) Diagnostic symptoms.

(b) Pathognomonic symptoms.

(c) Basic symptoms.

(d) Absolute symptoms.

(e) Generic symptoms.

(f) Pathological symptoms.
(g) Clinical symptoms.
(h) Local symptoms.
(i) Organic symptoms.

Stuart Close has clearly explained what is meant by the term common symptoms. He states that 'certain symptoms are selected as having known pathological relation to each other and upon these is based the diagnosis. The classification of symptoms thus made represents diagnostic idea.' The common symptoms are neither useful in differentiating a patient from another patient nor useful in differentiating various remedies from each other, therefore a true homeopathic prescription cannot be based on these symptoms.

> Degree of pathological changes a Degree of common symptoms.
> - Curability of disease.
> - Pathognosis.
> - Removal of maintaining causes.

Common Symptoms are considered as unimportant from homeopathic point of view but an observant physician can know many things about the case by taking note of the common symptoms too. More the number of common symptoms in the case more the pathological changes and lesser the chances of cure. The degree of pathological changes is directly proportional to the degree of common symptoms in the case. Higher potencies and certain deep acting drugs are contraindicated if there are advanced pathological changes in the case. The common symptoms although unimportant in prescribing can serve as a guide to physician in knowing the curability of the case. Thus, by observing the common symptoms physician is in a position to advice the patient about prognosis and measures necessary to remove the maintaining causes.

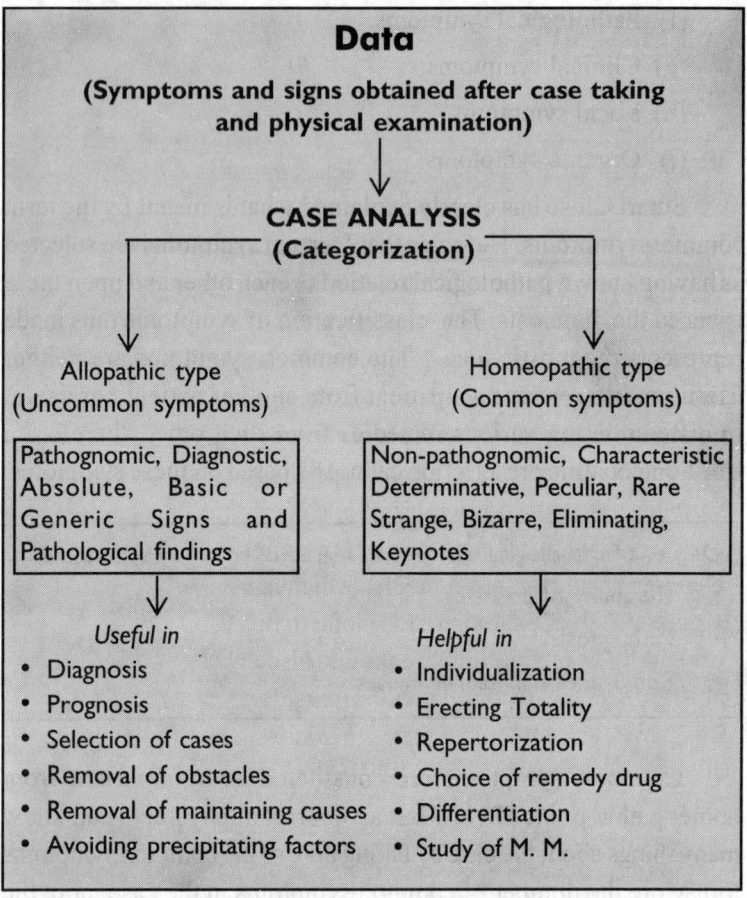

2. UNCOMMON AND CHARACTERISTIC SYMPTOMS

The word characteristic means 'a distinguishing quality.' The characteristics differentiate one patient from another and one remedy from the other. The symptoms that cannot be explained on the basis of pathology or diagnosis are called as uncommon or characteristic symptoms. All great homeopaths have repeatedly emphasized importance of uncommon symptoms or characteristic symptoms in homeopathic practice. It is because the characteristics refer to the patient as a whole and make the patient stand out from others suffering from the same disease. Patient's individuality gets expressed through what is uncommon in him. Patient calls for a specific remedy through the characteristics he presents with. A homeopath therefore is interested in what is uncommon in the case. Whole therapeutic programme depends upon uncommon symptoms or characteristic symptoms. Perhaps the key to successful homeopathic practice lies in the ability to perceive the characteristic in the patient and the remedy. Totality making, individualisation, study of materia medica, repertorisation, choice of remedy and almost all the other procedures carried out before the treatment of the patient are dependent on the proper appreciation of characteristics in the case. A proper appreciation of characteristics involves identifying and eliminating diagnostic symptoms, while studying a patient and identifying and comparing the characteristics produced by different remedies especially comparing the characteristics of those remedies which have similar pathogenesis. Appreciation of characteristics done in this manner makes the job of searching for simillimum easy and also enhances the physician's ability to perceive the patient's image and differentiate various images in homeopathic materia medica. Characteristic symptoms are like small dots and joining these dots reveals the patient's image as well as the remedy image in materia medica. A peculiar combination of characteristics constitutes the totality and provides individuality to the case. Following types of symptoms fall under the category of uncommon or characteristic symptoms:

(a) Guiding symptoms.
(b) Keynotes.
(c) Peculiar symptoms.
(d) Strange symptoms.
(e) Non-pathognomic symptoms.
(f) Determinative symptoms (Boericke).
(g) Rare and bizarre symptoms.

(h) Eliminating symptoms.

(i) Prescribing symptoms.

(j) Alternating symptoms.

(k) Qualified mentals.

(l) Attendent symptoms (Concomitants).

(m) Characteristic generals (including negative and pathological generals).

Some of the highly characteristic symptoms of a remedy are also called as keynotes by many and prescribing on keynotes has been strongly criticised by many since Hahnemann's time. Paradoxically these so called keynotes serve as basis for comparison of remedies. H.C. Allen in preface to first edition of 'Allen's Keynotes' comments on the value of keynotes by saying that, "It may be a so called 'keynote' a 'characteristic' the 'red strand of the rope' and central modality or principle as the aggravation from motion of *Bryonia alba,* the amelioration from motion of *Rhus,* the furious, vicious delirium of *Belladonna* or the apathetic indifference of *Phosphoric acid,* some familiar landmark around which the symptoms may be arranged in the mind for comparison." Stuart Close has very correctly defined 'Keynotes.' He states that, "A keynote may be defined as a concise statement of a single characteristic feature of a drug deduced by a critical consideration of its symptoms as recorded in proving or it is minor generalization based on study of particulars." He believes that 'keynote system' is strictly Hahnemannian. It is just that Dr. Guernesy has given a new name for old Hahnemannian idea of giving importance to characteristic symptoms. Keynote system has been criticized so much due to the tendency of some physicians to use single keynote for selection of remedy which is abuse of keynotes. To avoid pitfalls in use of keynotes for prescribing, Hering recommends that the prescription should be based on at least three or more characteristics or keynotes, provided generals are not contradicting the remedy suggested by keynotes. He calls it the 'three legged stool.'

Owing to the terminological inexactitude on part of some physicians and homeopathic authors the term 'peculiar symptom' is used synonymous to the term 'characteristic symptom.' However, it is important to understand that although a peculiar symptom is a characteristic symptom, but a characteristic symptom may not always be a peculiar symptom, because a peculiar symptom means a symptom that belongs exclusively to a particular remedy and none else. For example, stomach complaints of *Phos.* are ameliorated by cold drink and he craves cold water but it is vomited as soon as it gets warm in stomach; this is peculiar to ISimilarly coryza > by cold bathing is peculiar to *Calc. sulph.* While burning pains > by hot application is peculiar symptom of *Arsenicum album.*

A characteristic may belong to a group of remedies but a peculiar symptom is not a common property of a group of remedies and belongs solely to one remedy. Similarly, strange symptoms also fall under the category of characteristic symptoms. A strange symptom means a 'surprising unexpected characteristic' for example asthma is usually < by lying down but in a *Psorinum* patient asthma is > by lying down; this is unusual and surprising and hence a strange symptom of *Psorinum*. Similarly, stool passes easier when standing is a strange symptom of *Causticum* and *Alumina*. It must be always remembered that the more characteristic a symptom, lesser is the number of remedies it qualifies for final differentiation.

Generals and Particulars

The uncommon symptoms are further classified into two major classes Generals and Particulars. Generals relate to patient as a whole while the particulars relate to parts.

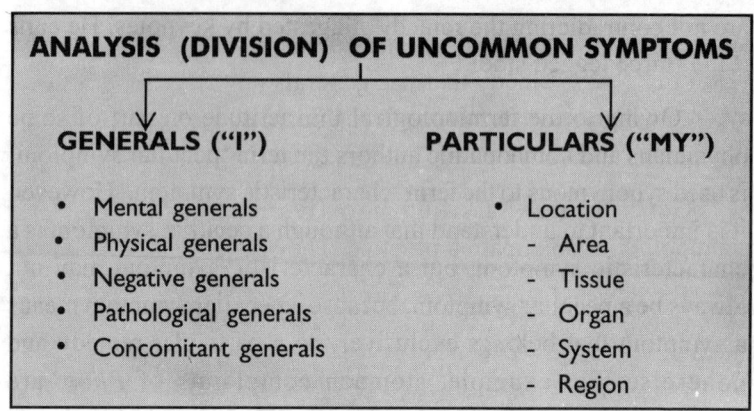

GENERALS

Generals form the outline of the case and generals give individuality to the case. In spite of the fact that generals represent the whole man, one need not forget that generals can be common too, and common generals such as weakness or languor during fever, loss of appetite during fever need to be eliminated from consideration while prescribing. Amongst the generals 'very characteristic generals' are the symptoms that cannot be omitted and form the essence of the individual. Generals are more important in chronic prescribing, while characteristic particulars assume importance in acute prescribing. Lack of skill in case taking makes the case record deficient in mental and physical generals and leads to abundance of particulars. A case record full of diagnostic and characteristic particulars but having no generals is what can be called 'an empty case record.' Such case record fails to be of use for scientific homeopathic prescribing.

Boenninghausen fully aware of difficulties involved in obtaining generals during case taking put forth the concept of 'generalization.' According to him, a symptom expressed in multiple locations can be safely categorized as a general symptom. Although Kent strongly criticized generalization, but he too has stressed on importance of generals in his lectures by saying that, "Don't expect a remedy that has generals must have all the little symptoms. It is a waste of time to run out all the little symptoms if the remedy has the generals."

Generals are classified into five main types from the standpoint of homeopathic practice. They are:
1. Mental Generals.
2. Physical Generals.
3. Negative Generals.
4. Pathological Generals.
5. Concomitant Generals.

1. MENTAL GENERALS

All great homeopaths repeatedly emphasized the importance of mentals. Keeping a psychosomatic perspective is must for

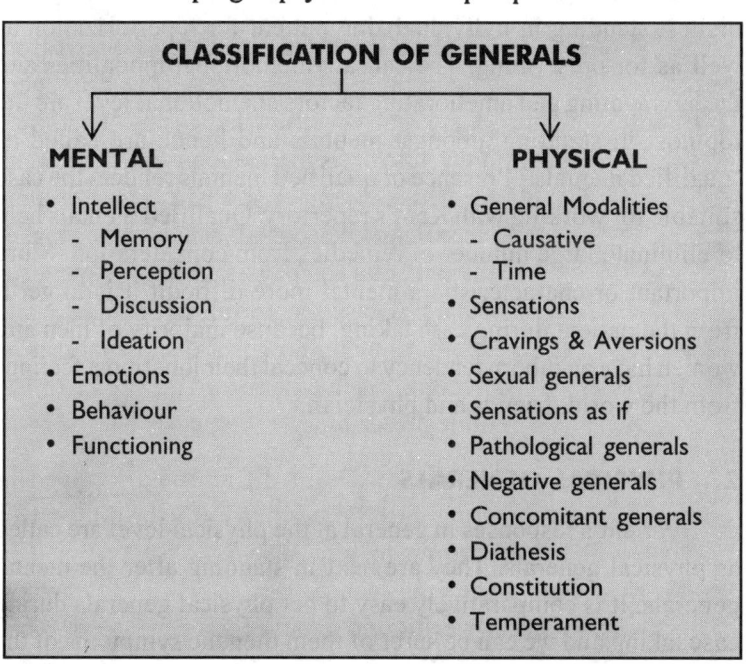

qualitative appreciation of an individual, which is necessary in homeopathic prescribing. Kent has rightly said that mentals represent the inner man and Stuart close states, "The mind is the man." This is because we are known by our actions. Actions in turn are the result of our own thoughts, feelings and desires. The essence of an individual therefore lies in his thoughts, feelings and desires which we call the mentals. Mentals are always expressed in general terms and cannot be expressed in terms like, "my hand is sad" or "My chest is angry" etc. and hence they express the man himself and not his parts and therefore they are classified as general symptoms. Among the mental generals the emotions, will, loves and hates, fears and anxieties and the causative emotional modalities are of higher value as compared to symptoms of intellect such as loss of memory and forgetfulness, etc.

Mentals form major portion of what is called the individualizing or personification of remedies. Mentals have highest standing in individualizing patient for repertorization as well as for prescribing. The causative emotional modalities and the aggravating and ameliorating factors at emotional level are the topmost in standing amongst mentals and hence are called as 'qualified mentals.' Presence of qualified mentals renders the case suitable for working with Kent's repertory. Qualified mentals help to eliminate large number of remedies from consideration. More important or characteristic a mental more difficult it is to get it from the patient during case taking, because majority of men and women have an inborn tendency to conceal their innermost feelings from the world, friends and physician.

2. PHYSICAL GENERALS

Patient's responses in general at the physical level are called as physical generals. They are next in standing after the mental generals. It is comparatively easy to get physical generals during case taking and we can be surer of them then the symptoms of the mind, hence Boenninghausen emphasized them in his repertory. All the general sensations and complaints at the physical level, recent deviations from psycho-physio-biological drives and norms and all the sensations as if come under the category of physical generals. Terms such as constitution, temperament and diathesis are always used to refer to the generalities of the physical type. General responses to physical, chemical, biological and physiological environment are to be considered as physical general modalities. Apart from physical reactions in general to the environment, the cravings, aversions, sweats in general, disturbances in sleep, dreams, disturbances in sexual sphere and aggravations noticed in relation to menstrual cycle are the responses to be considered as physical generals. Causative generalities include suppressions, vaccinations, miasms, and hereditary influences. The predisposing and precipitating causes are very beautifully given in the form of aggravating and ameliorating modalities in Boenninghausen's Therapeutic Pocket Book and are often useful for taking 'physical general modalities' as rubrics during repertorization and prescribing.

With regards to physical generals one thing should be always kept in mind that, whenever a modality or sensation is experienced in more than two locations it could be safely generalized. According to Boenninghausen a sensation or a modality with sufficient intensity can be taken from a complete symptom in the case and generalized which is second criteria for generalization.

3. NEGATIVE GENERALS

In some cases absence of certain customary or expected feature of a disease may be a general symptom of the case and such generals which are characterized by such peculiar absence are called as negative generals. For example, fever without thirst, coldness with aversion to being covered, dry mouth without thirst, asthma and arthritis not aggravated by cold, etc.

4. PATHOLOGICAL GENERALS

Prescribing on pathological basis is against the homeopathic doctrine, as homeopathy believes that disease makes itself known through symptoms and hence prime importance should be given to symptoms in prescribing especially to characteristic symptoms.

But considering the present day advances in diagnostic instruments we can see that disease makes itself known through pathological changes also, for example pain in abdomen is the expression of disease but the tumor in abdomen is also equally an expression of disease and therefore in cases with advanced pathological changes where there is maximum possibility of non-availability of characteristics the only thing left to prescribe upon is the propensity and tendency to certain types of pathological changes. Considering these factors Dr. C.M. Boger introduced the concept of pathological generals. According to him, the general tendency and propensity to certain types of pathological changes come under the category of generals which he called 'Pathological Generals.' Or in other words, the pathological changes, which are predicative of a generalized disturbance in patient's economy can be termed as pathological generals. Pathological generals express the pathological changes in relation to constitution. Structural alterations common to two or more locations can be taken as pathological generals by way of generalization. In his repertory, we find large number of such generals under 'Sensations and complaints in general.' Examples of pathological generals are uric acid diathesis, hemorrhage, bloody discharges, warts, fibrous tissue etc. Dr. J.C. Burnett also held the view of giving consideration to pathological generals in cases with deficiency of other characteristics.

5. CONCOMITANT GENERALS

The seemingly unrelated generals, which coexist with the chief complaint can be termed as concomitant generals.

Concomitant generals can be mental generals or physical generals. Concomitant generals pointing to a deep acting constitutional remedy are expressed most of the times towards the end of acute illness managed by acute remedy. Concomitant mental generals are important in physical complaint while concomitant physical generals are important in mental complaint. For example, irritability with earache (*Cham.*), restlessness with most of the complaints (*Acon., Ars., Rhus-t.*), and special cravings and aversions during fever, thirstlessness during fever are all concomitant generals. The characteristic concomitant generals serve as short cuts in acute prescribing many a times.

PARTICULARS

The symptoms that relate to parts of the body are called as particulars. Patient uses 'My' while describing them. They are also known as local symptoms. The characteristics at the level of particulars are important in acute prescribing. In chronic prescribing strong characteristic particulars become important for doing finer differentiation of remedies, if the generals are weak. Common particulars help the physician in diagnosis by making him aware of the area, region, tissues, and system affected by the disease. Although location is the last thing to be considered in homeopathic prescribing, but in acute cases with paucity of symptoms, it may help a neophyte in indicating a particular group of remedies, i.e. the remedies which have got special affinity to the particular location involved in the disease for example, locations such as joints and muscular tissue draw our attention to certain group of remedies such as *Rhus-t., Bry., Arn., Led., Colch., Benzoic acid,* and *Kali-c.* etc. After a closer inquiry a physician can differentiate the group of remedies thus indicated. In cases with lack of generals, the characteristic particulars become useful for generalization, i.e. for drawing generals out of particulars.

CONCEPT OF EVALUATION IN PRACTICE

Analysis gives physician a classified list of symptoms he is concerned with, but the symptoms in the list become useful only after they are re-arranged logically. The logical re-arrangement is decided by judging the value or importance of each symptom and the symptoms are then arranged in the order of importance. Value of a symptom depends upon its degree of peculiarity. More unusual a symptom more important it is for the physician. True individuality of any remedy is known by rare, strange, peculiar symptom, which can be called the 'core' of the remedy. Similarly true individuality of the patient can only be perceived by recognizing the rare, strange, peculiar symptoms of the patient, and hence they deserve greater importance than other uncommon symptoms. Evaluation involves understanding the hierarchy of symptoms. It gives individuality to the case by way of organizing patient's responses or symptoms in a certain manner.

The typical organization of symptoms provided by their evaluation plays very important role in establishing similarity. That is why, a good evaluator eventually becomes a good prescriber. Evaluation is fitting the right blocks of the case in right place to enable the formation of a meaningful whole. Giving emphasis on single symptom and prescribing on single symptom as many thoughtlessly do must not be done to prevent errors in evaluation according to Stuart Close. There lies maximum risk of error in evaluation as proper evaluation depends upon physician's ability to give each symptom its due importance and ability to strike a balance by not putting undue importance on those symptoms which don't deserve it from homeopathic point of view. Boger has summarized the perplexity of evaluation by saying that, "In the abstract the same symptom may have the highest standing in one case and the lowest in the next case, all depending upon general outline of the case as delineated by the associated symptoms."

Correct evaluation of symptoms presupposes that the symptoms taken for evaluation are complete symptoms having all the elements required and have been properly interpreted before including them in the case-record during case taking. Many consider evaluation to be a part of repertorization process and only important for repertorization of case but they are mistaken. Evaluation is necessary before totality making and choice of remedy, whether one wants to repertorize the case or not, it does not matter. Dr. Margaret Tyler rightly states that, "Key to case lies in grading of symptoms. It economises labour without compromising results."

In formal homeopathic education we learn about the evaluation of symptoms described by various stalwarts. Inspite of the fact that each one differs from another's method of evaluation but the basics of evaluation are more or less common to all of them. All agree that uncommon a symptom the greater is its value, but the emphasis varies according to the philosophy each one follows in practice. Consequently, in actual application of concept of evaluation one is likely to get confused due to the differences that existed between them and the differing terminologies and methods of evaluation used by them and hence an integrated approach to evaluation is necessary.

Following facts about evaluation emerge from an integration and synopsis of all the viewpoints regarding evaluation of symptoms:

1. Complete symptoms are more important than incomplete symptoms.
2. Characteristics are more important than common symptoms.
3. Generals are more important than particulars because they form the outline of the case.
4. Amongst the generals, mental generals have a higher gradation as compared to physical generals, because mentals denote

the inner man and are highly individualizing and amongst the mentals qualified mentals are more important than other mentals.

5. In evaluation of physical generals, the physical general modalities get the top ranking followed by cravings and aversions, disturbances in sleep and sex function, dreams, while the pathological generals get the lowest position.

6. Modality is more important than sensation because modalities characterize the particulars. The general modalities are more important than particular modalities

7. Amongst the various types of modalities the causative modality has a greater value than aggravating modality, which in turn ranks higher than ameliorating modality.

8. Predisposing causes are important in chronic cases where as precipitating causes assume importance in acute cases.

9. Amongst the sensations the 'sensations as if' and sensations experienced with greater intensity have higher value than common sensations, which only help in diagnosis.

10. Sensations are higher in position to concomitants and locations.

11. Mental concomitants are important in physical complaint and physical concomitants are of value in mental complaint.

SYNTHESIS OF CASE

Synthesis is the last step in case processing. Analysis deals with identification of parts, which is followed by qualitative appreciation of parts (symptoms) through the process of evaluation, while synthesis is the process of forming a structure out of parts. Qualitative appreciation determines the place of various parts in the structure, and therefore it precedes the synthesis. The structure thus formed is known as *Conceptual Image* or in other words totality of symptoms. The individuality thus established through formation of structure is most essential for remedial diagnosis. But synthesis does not mean bringing together of parts in a haphazard manner but it is a process of making a pattern through peculiar weaving of parts. The same group of parts can give rise to various forms of images depending upon their typical arrangement. The order of arrangement of symptoms is important, it should match with the layout of symptoms in materia medica and repertories, then only one is able to compare the patient's image with various remedies to select a suitable remedy.

■

CHAPTER 8

The Art of Perceiving 'Totality'

- ❖ What is Totality? 177
- ❖ What is Patient's Image or Portrait? 178
- ❖ Totality—'A Homeopathic Diagnosis' 179
- ❖ Prerequisites for Perceiving Totality 180
- ❖ Clincial Implications 181
- ❖ Method of Erecting Totality 183
- ❖ Tips for Clinical Judgement of Totality 187
- ❖ Illustrative Case 188

CHAPTER 8

THE ART OF PERCEIVING 'TOTALITY'

The information recorded in the case taking after being scrutinized or processed, is followed by erecting or rather perceiving the totality of symptoms. Once the case processing is done the physician gets a clear idea about the relative value of various symptoms in the case and how they are interlinked, so he is in a better position to perceive totality. Let us see what is totality and how to perceive the totality?

WHAT IS TOTALITY?

Symptoms are the expressions of the diseased individual.

The totality is:

- Recognizable pattern of characteristic expressions.
- Quantity of certain qualities.

The essence of these expressions which represents a patient's 'peculiar' or individual responsiveness at the level of mind and body is the totality or in other words totality is the recognizable pattern of expressions. The expressions or symptoms are made recognizable due to certain characteristic or individualizing features and therefore totality can be called as 'recognizable pattern of characteristic expressions.' Being dependent on characteristics, totality is a qualitative concept. It won't be wrong to say that it is the quantity of certain qualities, which together contribute to make an identifiable whole, which we know by the term 'Totality'.

WHAT IS PATIENT'S IMAGE OR 'PORTRAIT'?

Totality is often referred to as an 'Image' or 'Portrait' in homeopathic philosophical texts. Have we ever wondered, why it is called an image or portrait? The answer is simple. Totality consists of symptoms (characteristics). Symptoms are born from whatever a patient describes to the physician and whatever the physician observes in the patient. Thus symptoms are the existing facts on which totality or patient's image is constructed. One should note that although patient's image is based on facts it is not a concrete reality in itself. An image or portrait is an idea or a mental abstraction. It does not exist in the patient, but gets formed in physician's mind. It is the picture that emerges in the physician's mind after he conceptualizes the facts, with the help of analysis and evaluation as tools. That is why totality is often referred to as the portrait or the conceptual image of the patient. Remember that clinically it is a concept which helps in identifying the individual and the remedy needed to cure him. Symptoms are the only evidence of totality, through them it gets expressed. It is not visible but it has to be conceived and perceived through characteristics in the patient, by the physician. For example we can't see air but we have the evidences of its presence through movement of leaves and its other effects on the environment and from this knowledge comes the concept of air not visible but recognizable through its effects. So is totality a concept, which we recognize through study of characteristic expressions in a patient and the way in which they co-exist. Totality therefore is nothing but a conceptual image, formed out of a peculiar combination of characteristics which makes a patient unique.

TOTALITY - A 'HOMEOPATHIC DIAGNOSIS'

The response to the same stimulus varies from individual to individual and each individual response varies from another due to its own set of components and the arrangement of components.

Each individual has his own genetic makeup, hereditary background, type of susceptibility and physical makeup and therefore two individual responses to same disease stimulus can never be the same and hence the homeopathic stimulus (similar remedy) also has to be in accordance with the special type of

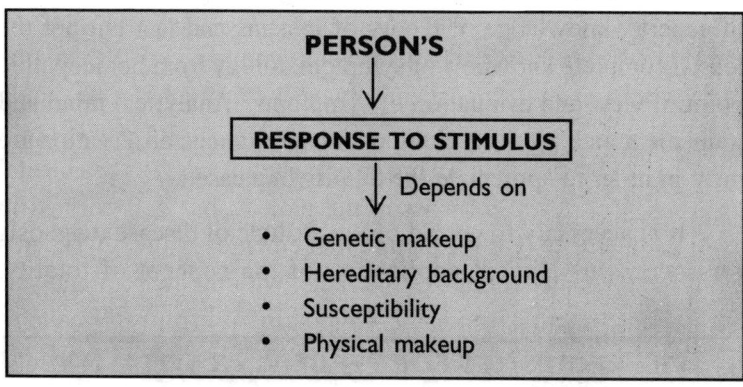

response exhibited by each individual; owing to this five patients suffering from disease of the same name are treated by five different remedies although they are suffering from the same disease. The remedies prescribed to them are chosen on the basis of unique totality seen in each one of them. Homeopathic practice is therefore 'individual specific.' The individualization which results from appreciation and application of concept of 'totality of symptoms,' is nothing but 'homeopathic diagnosis.' Therefore from practical point of view we can conclude that, "A homeopath diagnoses individuals suffering from diseases while an 'allopath' diagnoses diseases affecting the individual." This must be the guiding thought while prescribing if a homeopath wishes to be scientific in his approach to homeopathic practice. Hence, if the physician fails in this homeopathic diagnosis he is bound to fail in giving right homeopathic treatment. Greater our ability to comprehend totality greater is our ability to treat patients efficiently.

PREREQUISITES FOR PERCEIVING TOTALITY

The construction of totality or the ability to perceive totality demands the physician to have knowledge of homeopathic philosophy, clinical medicine, pathology, and psychology (normal and abnormal). It also requires knowledge of logic and philosophy in general, knowledge of theory of miasms and last but not the least a complete knowhow of symptomatology from homeopathic point of view and evaluation of symptoms. Analytical mind and judgement making skills along with unprejudiced observation are must in order to appreciate the totality of a case.

It is necessary to get rid of the attitude of disease diagnosis for successful clinical application of the concept of totality.

PRE REQUISITES FOR PERCEIVING TOTALITY

- Analytical mind
- Judgement skill
- Unprejudiced observation

Knowledge of:
- Homeopathic philosophy
- Clinical medicines
- Pathology
- Psychology
- Logic
- General philosophy
- Theory of miasms
- Development of symptoms homeopathically
- Evaluation of symptoms
- Psychology

Physician's thought process while constructing totality must be 'homeopathic' in the truest sense, where the 'individual' is more important than the disease or the pathology involved. Physician's ability to appreciate totality depends upon his ability to appreciate the language of symptoms through analysis and evaluation of symptoms.

The major obstacles in understanding the language of symptoms are non-observation, mal-observation and over generalization and misinterpretation of symptoms. Successful analysis and evaluation is a must to discover the totality of symptoms.

CLINICAL IMPLICATIONS

Hahnemannian philosophy can be described in just a single word 'totality,' and the one who has not understood this concept has not understood Hahnemann. Concept of totality is the 'heart of homeopathic practice.' Kent rightly calls it, 'The first principle of prescribing.' It is interesting to note that the word 'Totality' appears in as many as 27 aphorisms in the Organon of Medicine and that is a sufficient proof of the high degree of emphasis laid on it by Hahnemann. This is because the concept of totality represents the final synthesis of the mental process carried out by the physician with respect to the patient. It embraces the whole homeopathic doctrine.

As already stated the ability to see the totality depends upon the ability to analyze and evaluate symptoms, but this is only partially true. It must never be forgotten that the knowledge of totalities of the drugs is equally important for clinical perception of totality, because the concept of totality incorporates both the patient and the remedy. To know a patient is to know his individuality that is represented by his totality, similarly to know a drug is to know it in its totality, cure results from coming together of the two totalities. Our memory recognizes only that which it knows and hence only when we know the drug totalities, we would be able to recognize them in our patients. The high degree of clarity in understanding drug totalities is the only thing that can prevent us from finding different remedial agents for the same patient. Every drug has its own distinct individuality, its own totality; this must be kept in mind. Knowing this fact is the first step towards successful clinical application of the concept of totality.

The totality should be such that it differentiates the patient in question from other patient suffering from disease of same name and thereby results in employment of a different remedy from that prescribed to the other patient, but this does not happen inspite of our best efforts when the totality of symptoms is seen as a 'list of characteristics,' but exactly there lies the greatest conceptual error. Totality is never a mere list of characteristics but it is the typical way in which the characteristics in the list co-exist. A mere list of characteristics can indicate 2 or 3 remedies but when the pattern of co-existence is understood we reach to only one remedy out of the 2 or 3 remedies. Hence the 'typical form of co-existence' is the soul of the concept of totality, as this form of co-existence is responsible for converting a mere list of characteristic into an image or portrait of the patient and, therefore a physician must strive to see this soul in every case whether acute or chronic.

But a physician would like to know how to comprehend the pattern of characteristics in every case? Farrington has already given the solution to this while describing the true value of totality by saying that every characteristic has to be measured by its relation to the whole to understand the whole. Pattern is that element of the whole which is seen in all its parts. A pattern is known by the common string that runs through all the parts of it. Similarly, 'Pattern of characteristics' is the resultant of logical generalization of particulars. For example, Clarke while describing *Cantharis vesicatoria* in his 'Dictionary of Materia Medica', says that, "The word "irritation" best expresses the totality of the *Cantharis* effects," Kent while describing *Bryonia* states that, "Thus we have the well-known *Bryonia alba* aggravation from motion. This runs all through the remedy." What they wanted to say is that we can make out *Bryonia alba* from < motion and we can identify *Cantharis vesicatoria* by the irritation, because these features are seen through the length and breadth of these drugs. Similarly, knowing the patient's totality is knowing those peculiarities which represent the patient as a whole or those peculiarities which express themselves from every side and every angle of the case.

METHOD OF ERECTING TOTALITY

The logical arrangement of characteristics (according to order of importance) constitutes totality. Only the characteristic expressions present in the state of illness can never constitute a totality. Totality is essentially an evolutionary, qualitative and dynamic concept. Totality being an evolutionary phenomenon the time dimension comes in to picture. Perceiving totality in true sense therefore demands, taking into consideration the total span of time over which the phenomenon of disease occurs from past to present, with possible projections into future.

This means that in clinical practice after recording the case a physician should examine in full detail the manner in which an individual has evolved. The phases through which he has passed and the manner in which he has met the surroundings (environment) to produce the 'individualized illness response.' To do this physician should take into account:

1. The principle of causation.
2. The principle of concomitance.
3. The knowledge of evolution.

4. The determination of phases.

A patient evolves from a healthy person into a diseased individual. Evolution means change taking place from time to time. Therefore, a physician is also expected to pay attention to:

(i) The rate of change.

(ii) The direction of change.

(iii) The levels of involvement.

(iv) The area of involvement.

CONSIDERATIONS WHILE ERECTING TOTALITY

- The principle of causation.
- The principle of concomitance.
- The knowledge of evolution.
  - The rate of change.
  - The direction of change.
  - The levels of involvement.
  - The area of involvement.
- The determination of phases.

Knowledge of various components or constituents of the conceptual image and their order of arrangement in the portrait is important for construction of conceptual image or patient's totality.

The core of the image consists of causative factors, both predisposing as well as precipitating. The precipitating emotional as well as physical factors are often referred to as 'Ailments from.' Among them emotional factors get a higher place in construction of conceptual image. The predisposing factors are important in chronic cases, because they make the individual susceptible to various illnesses. They are also responsible for frequent relapses. The predisposing factors include diathesis, temperament, hereditary influences, miasms, suppressions and vaccination.

Second in the order are general modalities both mental and physical. They provide form to the image. Among the general modalities, those circumstances that aggravate the chief complaint as well as the concomitant are all important. The individualizing general characteristics at mental and physical level, which portray the individual to the physician, are placed next in the logical arrangement of totality. Among the mental characteristics, manifestations of disturbed feeling state like anger, sadness, fear, and impulsive behaviour deserve greater importance than those of intellectual sphere like disturbances of memory, perception, formulation and discrimination.

Last but not the least are the characteristics at particular level. Especially the particulars that are peculiar, queer, rare and strange. These particulars very often prove helpful in pinpointing the remedy. But, according to Dr. Kent, if the remedy is clearly indicated by other features of the case one should not insist on matching every little particular in the case. Even if the particulars do not correspond, clinical experience has shown that the remedy acts in a curative manner.

The definite plan consisting of various heading under which the analysed data needs to be arranged for evolving an individual image of the patient is given below:

1. CAUSATION
    (i) Fundamental Cause (miasmatic).
    (ii) Disposition.
    (iii) Precipitating Factors:
        (a) Emotional.
        (b) Physical.

```
┌─────────────────────────────────────────────┐
│         CHARACTERISTIC PARTICULARS          │
│           • Modalities                      │
│           • Sensations                      │
│           • Concomitants                    │
│           • Location         ▼              │
│  ┌────────────────────────────────────────┐ │
│  │   Sensations & Complaints in General   │ │
│  │           • Mental                     │ │
│  │           • Physical                   │ │
│  │  ┌──────────────────────────────────┐  │ │
│  │  │ Circumstances of Agg. & Amel. in │  │ │
│  │  │              General             │  │ │
│  │  │        • Emotional               │  │ │
│  │  │        • Physical                │  │ │
│  │  │  ┌────────────────────────────┐  │  │ │
│  │  │  │ Causation:                 │  │  │ │
│  │  │  │   • Fundamental cause      │  │  │ │
│  │  │  │   • Disposition            │  │  │ │
│  │  │  │   • Precipitating factors  │  │  │ │
│  │  │  │      • Emotional           │  │  │ │
│  │  │  │      • Physical            │  │  │ │
│  │  │  └────────────────────────────┘  │  │ │
│  │  └──────────────────────────────────┘  │ │
│  └────────────────────────────────────────┘ │
└─────────────────────────────────────────────┘
```

2. Circumstances of Aggravation and Amelioration in general.
   (i) Emotional (Mental).
   (ii) Physical.
3. Sensations and Complaints in general.
   (Mental and physical characteristics of the patient)
4. Characteristic Particulars
   (i) Modalities (Causative, <, >, Peculiar, Strange).
   (ii) Sensations ("Sensation as if").
   (iii) Concomitants.
   (iv) Location (Part, Area of spread).

It is not necessary that one would find all these features in every case in practice. The above plan serves as a guide to a novice, who may not be as gifted as the intuitive prescriber who prescribes just after a single glance at the case record. The arrangement of characteristics in totality may vary from case to case. This is because the facts collected in each case are different. However the golden rule in totality construction is that, features of the case which are greater in value are placed at the top followed by less important features.

TIPS FOR CLINICAL JUDGEMENT OF TOTALITY

1. Concentrate on what is uncommon in the case; don't get overwhelmed by the quantity of symptoms, laboratory investigation & x-ray reports of the case.
2. Remember, the distant you are from diagnostic signs & symptoms and tissue changes the closer you are to totality.
3. Be alert and remember totality does not always result from what patient tells you but may result from what you observe in the patient.
4. If a patient comes from other homeopathic physician don't forget to thoroughly go through the earlier physician's case record as it may reveal to you what you have missed while constructing the patient's totality.
5. If your patient returns to you after a long time, study the patient afresh, avoid the temptation to judge his totality on his previous record because his totality may have changed this time from what it was earlier.
6. Each symptom has to be judged keeping in mind the patient concerned with regards to how uncommon it is. For example, 'Craving for meat' is very common in certain non-vegetarian

7. A balance in trusting & suspecting the patient is must while collecting data. Trust as much as you can but also learn to suspect so that the truth is revealed to you.
8. Greatest error in making totality results from putting too much emphasis on single component of patient's symptoms either mental or physical.
9. Concentrate on those characteristics which repeatedly express themselves at all the levels.
10. Never forget that totality is a portrait of the patient and not just a list of characteristics.

ILLUSTRATIVE CASE
(Perceiving Totality and Remedy selection: Non-repertorial approach)

An unmarried girl aged 25 years, complains of dry^{2+}, maculo-papular, whitish, $itching^{2+}$ eruptions on face especially cheeks, chin and neck since last 3 years. Complaints were ameliorated for a short period by allopathic treatment, homeopathy from other physicians didn't help and it aggravated the problem. She has left it since past 1 month.

The skin complaints especially itching is aggravated by

- Washing face
- After $bathing^{3+}$
- Summer and heat of sun^{3+}
- Sour things
- $Soaps^{3+}$
- $Ointments^{3+}$
- Perspiration
- Damp $weather^{2+}$
- Change of $weather^{2+}$
- Drafts of air
- When she covers the face with $hankerchief^{2+}$ (while driving)

communities, but if seen in a Brahmin or any other community known to be strictly vegetarian it becomes most uncommon.

Amelioration by vaseline application.

Itching with blackish discolouration on neck is aggravated by wearing metallic jewellery²⁺.

Also since last 2 years, there has been recurrent cough and breathlessness with thick greenish expectoration; aggravated in damp weather²⁺, change of weather²⁺, morning, bathing, lying down, walking and ameliorated by sitting²⁺.

- **Built**: She is thin, having wheatish complexion, grey eyes and dry skin in general
- **Height**: 5.2 inches
- **Weight**: 42 kg
- **Desires**: Sour²⁺, boiled eggs²⁺, salt²⁺, sweets, spicy and pungent things
- **Aversion**: Milk²⁺
- **Bowels**: Regular
- **Urine**: No urinary complaints
- **Sweat**: Scanty, especially on head, arms and lower limbs; non-staining and without odour
- **Appetite**: Satisfactory
- **Thirst**: Less
- **Sleep**: She has light sleep broken by least noise. Sleep is unrefreshing. Sometimes wakes up at 1pm and cannot go to sleep again.
- **Dreams**: She has fearful dreams²⁺ of snakes²⁺, of somebody running after her, of dead bodies and of dead people.
- **Thermal Reaction**: She prefers bathing in luke warm water throughout the year except summer. She wants fanning through out the year³⁺. She is averse to covering

on legs[3+] and covers in general[3+], covers are required only in winter. She prefers warm food and drink. Rainy weather aggravates associated complaints. She feels severe heat and burning in legs and soles and to relieve it she has to take wet sheet on legs or dip them in cold water, this happens more frequently in summer. Sometimes she has headache from being in sun for long. Moist cooler air causes slight body ache and sneezing.

There is a past history of typhoid, malaria and jaundice. In childhood, she suffered from worms and recurrent tonsillitis. Her mother has arthritis and father has eczema. Also, there is family history of diabetes and high blood pressure. Maternal grandmother has recurrent respiratory complaints.

- **Menarche**: 13 years
- **Frequency**: Regular
- **Duration**: 5 days
- **Quantity**: Moderate
- **Colour**: Bright red with few clots, sometimes brownish colour. Stains are washable, odour is offensive.
- **Pain**: She has lumberache before menses but it is bearable.
- No complaints during and after menses.

She has one younger sister, presently graduating with science.

She has been an irritable child and had an obstinate childhood. She is more inclined to her father as he is of a mild nature (sober temper), whereas her mother keeps scolding her and pointing out her flaws and mistakes. Mother is irritable. She cannot bear anything happening against her wishes, she thinks everything must happen according to her wishes, never satisfied until her wish is completed. According to her, her sister is liked more in the family inspite of the fact that she can do everything that her sister is doing. In college she takes part in extra curricular activities like music, singing, drama, etc. At present she has joined music classes. She is an extrovert and mixes easily with anybody. Her academic achievements are mediocre. She passed with 51% in SSC and 60% in HSC. She justifies her scoring less in SSC due to a love affair.

They were going smoothly for some years but one day she got angry on him as the boy was not behaving properly and broke the relationship. Since this happened she has become more irritable. She still remembers him and broods over the past (time spent with him). She has been sad and depressed since that time. She wept a lot for some months after they broke up. She feels that even now she has not come out of it fully. She can't tolerate domination by anyone and gets severely angry. If anyone insults her she never keeps any contact with that person even if he apologizes afterwards. If she gets angry on anyone, she never forgets and teaches him a lesson at a suitable time later. Patient says that by nature she is an angry person and perhaps that is her biggest fault. She can't control her anger although sometimes she repents for being so angry. These days she gets irritated over trifles and vents her fury often. She is about to get married and she is worried about her irritable nature if this continues it would be difficult for her to adjust her self with her husband and in-laws when she gets married.

Mother often tells her to control her anger but she can't although she knows it is not good for her. Whenever she gets angry she trembles and has palpitation, face becomes red and hot and has a hatred feeling for the person with whom she is quarrelling. She is averse to doing any housework unless and until mother forces her to do it. Her mother keeps on asking her for one work after another and this makes her irritated. If her mother forces her too much she doesn't do anything. Her younger sister is presently engaged with a boy, she tells her sister to avoid contact with the boy and end the relationship as it would hurt her (sister), but the sister does not listen to her and so she sometimes gets irritated. She is fearful and anxious while on the road, fears accidents.

Sometimes feels somebody is coming to hurt her. She feels that her ex-boyfriend would follow her and hurt her. She thinks so as there are frequent news items of such incidents in newspapers. These days wants to be alone in house but fears when she is alone. She can't sleep near open window thinks that somebody would come from the window and kill her. Sometimes she has a strange idea while sleeping that the ceiling fan would fall on her as it has been loose since few months and makes noises. Feels jealous about her friends who score better marks and who are better than her in extracurricular activities. She was quiet worried about her skin complaints and homeopathy was suggested by an acquaintance. She feels she should get relieved fast with homeopathic treatment as she is going to get married next month.

Physical Examination:

- Pulse: 72/min
- BP: 120/80 mm of Hg
- Tongue: Clean
- Nails: Normal
- Conjunctiva: Normal

CASE WORKING

DIFFERENTIAL DIAGNOSIS

1. **Contact Dermatitis**: Patient complains of itching, dry blackish skin eruptions on neck and face aggravated by soaps, ointments, wearing metallic jewellery and by washing face. These clinical features are characteristic of contact dermatitis.

2. **Chronic infective bronchitis:** Patient complains of recurrent cough and breathlessness with thick greenish expectoration aggravated by change of weather, go in favour

of bronchitis (Cough for 2 consecutive years for at least 3 months duration). The mucopurulent discharges suggest presence of infection.

ASSESSMENT OF THERMALITY

No.	Description	Hot	Ambithermal	Chilly
1	Prefers bathing with luke warm water throught the year except summer.	√		
2	She wants fanning through out the year^{3+}.	√		
3	She is averse to covering on legs^{3+} and covers in general^{3+}	√		
4	She prefers warm food and drink.			√
5	She feels severe heat and burning in legs and soles and to relieve it she has to take wet sheet on legs or dip them in cold water this happens more frequently in summer.	√		
6	Sometimes she has headache from being in sun for long.	√		
7	< Summer and heat of sun^{3+} Chief Complaints.	√		
8	< When she covers the face with hankerchief^{2+} - Chief Complaints.	√		

No.	Description	Hot	Ambithermal	Chilly
9	Moist cooler air causes slight body ache and sneezing.			√
10	< Change of weather^{2+}- Associated complaints		√	

From the above table we can conclude that the patient is HOT^{3+}

INTERPRETATION OF MENTAL STATE

Inellect	Mediocre
Emotions	Anger^{3+} Anxiety^{3+} Fear
Behaviour	Quarrelsome Obstinate Timid
Functioning	Indolent
Expressions	Anger Hatred Anxiety Fear of someone approaching of being alone Suspicion Mistrust Jealousy Sadness Depression Grief

TOTALITY OF SYMPTOMS

Family History
- Diabetes
- High blood pressure
- Arthritis
- Eczema
- Respiratory complaints

Past History
- Typhoid
- Malaria
- Jaundice
- Worms
- Tonsillitis

Mental State
- Inellect – Mediocre
- Emotions – Anger[3+]
- Anxiety[3+]
- Fear
- Behaviour – Quarrelsome
- Obstinate
- Timid
- Functioning – Indolent

Thermality
Hot Patient[3+]

Generals (Modalities)
- < Covers^{3+}
- < Summer^{3+}
- < Bathing

Mental Generals (Sensations)
- Anger
- Hatred
- Anxiety
- Fear of someone approaching
- Being alone
- Suspicion
- Mistrust
- Jealousy
- Sadness
- Depression
- Grief

Physical Generals (Sensations)

Dreams: Fearful^{2+}, snakes^{2+}, dead people, dead bodies

Sleep: Unrefreshing, wakes up at 1pm. Can't go to sleep again

Cravings: Salt^{2+}, sours^{2+}, boiled eggs

Spicy: Pungent things, sweets

Aversion: Milk^{2+}

Thirst: Diminished

Sweats: Scanty

CHARACTERISTIC PARTICULARS

1. Eruption Face and Neck
- < Summer^{3+}
- < Bathing^{3+}
- < Heat of sun^{3+}
- < Soaps^{3+}
- < Ointments
- < Metal Jewellery^{3+}
- < Covering^{2+}
- < Change of weather^{2+}
- < Damp weather^{2+}
- < Drafts^{2+}
- < Washing
- Dry^{2+}
- Itching^{2+}

2. Cough, Breathlessness, Respiratory System
- < Damp weather^{2+}
- < Change of weather^{2+}
- < Morning
- < Bathing
- < Lying down
- < Walking
- > sitting^{2+}

3. < Before Menses
- Pain lumbar region

REMEDY SELECTION

The hot remedies that came up for consideration on the basis of above totality are Natrium muriaticum, Lycopodium clavatum, Lachesis mutus, Sulphur and Natrium sulphuricum.

Natrium sulphuricum was selected as the simillimum for this case due to its close correspondence to patient's totality. This patient reported amelioration of itching within one week of administering a single dose at bed time. The eruptions had subsided to a great extent by the end of second week. Facial skin returned to normalcy in another week. It need not be told that patient was much happier considering the fact that she was going to get married in the following month. The patient was under treatment for another year and a half. Her attacks of cough also reduced both in intensity as well as frequency.

■

CHAPTER 9

Scientific Approach to Repertorization

- ❖ Selection of Repertory for a Case   205
- ❖ Symptom to Rubric Translation   207
- ❖ Construction of Repertorial Syndrome   207
- ❖ Choice of Eliminating Symptoms   209
- ❖ Use of Cross-Repertorization   210
- ❖ Illustrative Case   213

CHAPTER 9

SCIENTIFIC APPROACH TO REPERTORISATION

Once the totality is constructed in accordance with the principles, the next important job is finding a suitable remedy. A well-made totality itself tells the remedy needed to establish similarity for cure in majority of cases. But sometimes in a case which is complicated one, the totality may not clearly indicate a single remedy and in such cases many remedies need to be thought of and compared before arriving at the perfect simillimum. Unfortunately, human memory falls too short of storing the vast homeopathic materia medica. Here comes the role of an assistant in the form of an instrument which takes care of storing and indexing the materia medica which we know by the name of repertory. Thus, in such cases repertorization becomes necessary. We know that repertorization is a process of arriving at a small group of indicated remedies for a particular case, mathematically with the use of a suitable repertory. But one common mistake is to consider repertorization to be only mathematics, which results from a mechanical approach to repertorization by neophytes and even by some experienced physicians.

Hahnemann was fully aware of the fact that too much dependence on repertories and casual approach to repertorization can lead to blunders in prescribing and hence just when the homeopathic repertory was in its childhood years, we find Hahnemann commenting on this aspect in his letter to Boenninghausen dated 26 December, 1834.

He writes, *"Even if the homeopathicians perceive that the repertories are insufficient for finding the best remedy for every case of disease, nevertheless they calm down when they have such an overview in their hands, and then believe (with some probability) to be able to dispense with the sources and don't buy and don't use them."*

Around 200 repertories have been published till now and many more are expected to come, but paradoxically with the increasing number of repertories the number of physicians using repertory mechanically & casually has also increased by leaps and bounds that is why we see many practitioners thumbing the repertory (Kent's Repertory majority of times) and trying to search a particular symptom or a disease condition and the remedy indicated for it. Some of them even prescribe a single remedy if the rubric has only one remedy mentioned in front of it. This very erroneous practice is most prevalent in present day homeopaths and neophytes. They fail to understand that repertory is only an instrument which tells what to prescribe. *Repertory only suggests while Materia Medica decides.* Such mechanical use of repertory produces horrible results and may prove very devastating to the patient's treatment.

A repertory is as good as the one who uses it. A repertory proves useless if the one who wishes to use it does not know how to use it. If used properly and scientifically it is a blessing. For judicious use of repertory and for deriving the maximum out of the process of repertorization one must be fully conversant with the underlying principles of repertorization. A routine repertorization is different from a scientific repertorization. Hence, a scientific approach to repertorization is must if one wants to get correct results out of this instrument. Artistic method and mechanical method are the two methods popularly described in majority of books on repertorization. It is said that the artistic method is more scientific and suitable for experienced physicians. It must be mentioned here that even the mechanical method must confirm to the tenets of science and thus should be as scientific as the so-called artistic method.

Repertorization like all other concepts in homeopathy is essentially a qualitative concept. It is a process where we proceed first from quality to quantity by studying the general list of drugs for a particular rubric or symptom and then from quantity to quality by going from a general list of drugs one proceeds to a particular group of indicated remedies which emerge during the process of repertorization by virtue of possessing the same qualities i.e. characteristics that a patient's totality indicates. This is progressive individualization. Repertorization is, therefore, the use of both the inductive and deductive logic where by we arrive at a conclusion from general to particular. Although repertorization is a mathematical process but homeopathy is not mathematics. Through repertorization we search for a probable group of 2-3 drugs for the numerical totality and as totality is not a numerical total of symptoms, materia medica must be the final court before a physician actually arrives at a simillimum. Therefore, the scientific repertorization is the logical use of the mathematical process of repertorization to minimize the number of remedies for final comparison to be done using materia medica.

One must not forget that materia medica contains the typical portrait of every individual drug formed by a typical pattern of its characteristics where as repertory contains symptoms which may be in a split form due to their conversion into rubrics and also the fact that repertory does not contain the characteristic symptoms only. As Dr. Kasad rightly puts it, "A repertory is mainly at general level, the homeopathic materia medica is at the level of specificity and fitness, which gets lost during transfer of symptoms to rubrics in the repertories." This makes it even more necessary to use a repertory with caution and scientificity to avoid blunders resulting from its injudicious use.

Incorrect translation of symptoms into rubrics, use of 'favourite repertory' for every case without giving consideration to the type of symptoms available for repertorization in a case, incorrect choice of symptoms for repertorization and the worst, incorrect choice of eliminating rubric are some of the most common mistakes which make the repertorization mechanical and unscientific.

ERRORS IN REPERTORIZATION RESULT FROM

- Poor evolution of the Generals during Case taking.
- Giving importance to symptoms of a low order.
- Generalization on inadequate grounds.
- Faulty symptom to rubric translation.
- Improper selection of eliminating symptom.
- Faulty repertory choice.

Scientific approach to repertorization involves:
1. Selection of repertory according to demands of the case and not on personal preferences.
2. Correct translation of symptoms into rubrics.
3. Logical application of the concept of Repertorial Syndrome.
4. Choice of eliminating symptom by judging the value of the symptom taken with reference to the case in hand.
5. Cross repertorization where necessary.

1. SELECTION OF REPERTORY FOR A CASE

The need for selecting a suitable repertory for every individual case arises from the fact that each repertory varies in its approach to repertorization as each one is based on different philosophical background. Each approach has its distinct scope of application and hence the most rewarding one for a given case must be selected. Similarly the content and the emphasis on particular type of rubrics also varies with every repertory. Hence, only a single repertory is suitable for a given case depending on the type of symptoms that dominate the totality and the type of case in hand.

Boenninghasuen's Therapeutic Pocket Book

Because of the generalization on grand scale and importance given to physical generals with special emphasis on concomitants Boenninghausen's Therapeutic Pocket Book is suitable for a case with well-marked physical generals especially the physical general modalities and cases with prominent concomitants and cases with prominent sensations and modalities in some parts but vague in other parts. It is most useful in cases which lack reliable mental symptoms and cases with paucity of symptoms in general.

Kent's Repertory

While Kent's repertory due to limited generalization, prime importance to mental generals and well-represented particulars is suitable for cases where well-marked and qualified mentals predominate the totality. It is also useful in cases with well-marked characteristic particulars. It can be more favourably used in cases where complete representation of each category of symptoms is available. Some cases are however suitable for both Boenninghausen's and Kent's repertory and doing so leads to identical results in the right hands.

Boger-Boenninghausen's Repertory

Boger's repertory due to the emphasis on pathological generals suits cases with predominance of pathological generals. Fever is well represented in Boger's repertory and hence it can be successfully used in cases of intermittent fever with well marked stages of chill, heat and sweat.

Synthetic Repertory

Generals both mental and physical are well represented in synthetic repertory which makes it suitable for cases with well represented generals but lacking in particulars of characteristic order. It cannot be used for acute cases where particulars dominate the picture.

Robin Murphy's Repertory

This repertory can be utilized for repertorizing all types of cases. (i.e. cases having prominent generals and / or particulars.) It is based on Kent's repertory. The chapters are arranged in alphabetical order. It follows three grades of remedies as suggested by Kent. Some additional chapters have been added that increase its utility from practical point of view. This repertory is suitable to cases where Kent's repertory can be used but the lack of rubrics is the obstacle in using Kent's Repertory. The seasonal modalities are very well represented in this repertory.

Clinical Repertories

Clinical repertories are not useful for scientific repertorization as they are based on diagnosis and pathological rubrics. These repertories can be used for reference purpose only in a case with advanced pathological changes and paucity of characteristics.

2. SYMPTOM TO RUBRIC TRANSLATION

Conversion of symptoms to rubrics is another important task which needs to be done very carefully and with precision, if one wants to execute the procedure of repertorization scientifically. Exact meaning of the symptom must be understood for correct translation of symptoms into rubrics. Knowing the arrangement of rubrics and the type of language in the repertory being used is also equally important. Misinterpretation of both the symptom and the rubric leads to distortion of the meaning and results in inexact list of drugs during repertorization.

3. CONSTRUCTION OF REPERTORIAL SYNDROME (RS)

A reportorial syndrome or reportorial totality consists of group of symptoms taken for actual repertorization on repertorization sheet or it is the essential totality used for the purpose of repertorization. Construction of reportorial syndrome is the most important part of repertorization process. Mechanical use of repertory always results from errors in construction of reportorial syndrome. Great caution, thoughtfulness and high degree of selectivity on part of the physician are required for proper construction of reportorial syndrome. Repertorial syndrome essentially consists of the generals of the case and it is only a part of patient's totality. Repertorial syndrome varies with the type of repertory, because a repertorial syndrome has to be framed in accordance with the logic applied i.e. the philosophical background of the repertory to be used.

Every repertory due to its typical approach and philosophy demands only certain type of symptoms to be included in the essential totality or repertorial totality, hence repertorial totality is variable and changes with the repertory used. A repertorial totality therefore consists of symptoms arranged according to hierarchy of importance depending upon the principles and logic of repertory used. The small group of symptoms remaining after deducing the reportorial totality from the conceptual image (i.e. totality of symptoms which forms the portrait of the patient) is known as 'potential differential field,' which should be taken into consideration for final differentiation of emerging remedies after the repertorization is done. Construction of repertorial syndrome without giving due consideration to the logic of repertory applied is unscientific way of repertorization and may prove damaging to the process of repertorization. Although the construction of reportorial syndrome primarily depends upon availability of data in every individual case, still some general guidelines can be given regarding construction of RS with various repertories which are as follows:

A reportorial totality of a case to be worked out by Kent's repertory will have qualified mentals at the top followed by physical generals and finally a few particulars if they are highly characteristic in the case. If the eliminating method is used the eliminating rubric should be put at the top.

While working with Boenninghausen's Therapeutic Pocket Book with the Robert's method the RS based on Boenninghausen's approach would have to be arranged in the order of modalities first followed by characteristic concomitants, sensations and finally the location. But when the case is repertorized by Dr. Dhawale's method then the reportorial or essential totality would have general modalities at the top followed by mental general sensations (mentals) and /or physical general sensations if they are very characteristic in the case.

When repertorizing with Boger-Boenninghausen's Complete Repertory (BBCR) if pathological generals are available in the case then they should be placed at the top considering the emphasis to pathological generals in BBCR. The pathological generals are to be followed by physical generals, concomitants and modalities. In a case where we have well marked causative modalities as well as other modalities, the causative modality would occupy the first position followed by aggravating modalities especially the time modalities and ameliorations and then the physical generals, concomitants and finally the location. The time modalities are to be taken prior to other modalities considering the importance given to them in BBCR.

A format of Repertorial Syndrome / Totality is given in **Appendix D** to aid the student physician. It would be of help for employing in both the academic institutions as well as in practice. The format is based on the one, which is commonly followed by majority of homeopathic physicians although individual variations may exist.

4. CHOICE OF ELIMINATING SYMPTOM

The drudgery and labour involved in the process of repertorization makes the short-cut of using eliminating rubric most popular amongst students, lecturers and physicians using Kent's repertory. The eliminating method is so popular that it has become synonymous with repertorization by Kent's repertory. We often forget that neither it is the only method of working cases with Kent's repertory, nor it is compulsory to repertorize every case with eliminating rubric. It needs to be emphasized here that the selection of eliminating symptom is a job that needs utmost care on part of the physician, because it is very crucial point of the case as only remedies indicated in this symptom are taken for repertorization thus if there is negligence in selection of eliminating symptom the likely remedy might get 'eliminated' from the list. Using eliminating rubric for repertorization is thus a 'risky short-cut.' The selection of eliminating symptom has to be governed by its importance in patient's totality to be scientific. Correct appreciation of the value and significance of a symptom in a case is must before selecting any symptom as eliminating symptom. It requires clinical depth and experience which a novice seldom has.

A qualitative evaluation of characteristics of the patient to select the eliminating symptom is only possible if the case is well-taken. This is not possible if the case lacks all the necessary data and hence use of eliminating method should be avoided if the case is not well recorded. When a single symptom doesn't seem valuable enough to be the eliminating one then two or three rubrics can be taken together as Dr. Margaret Tyler has recommended. Dr. Gibson Miller's idea of taking only chilly or hot remedies depending of patient's thermality leaves a chance of the most likely remedy being thrown out from the repertorization list and therefore is not advisable. Based on the logic behind the concept of eliminating symptom some basic rules for its selection can be formulated, which are as follows:

(i) The symptom selected should have such high rank in the totality, that it can never be omitted while searching the simillimum for the case.

(ii) A highly characteristic general is always preferable.

(iii) Qualified mentals especially a causative emotional modality can be safely selected as eliminating symptom.

(iv) A strong characteristic general which expresses any constitutional peculiarity of the patient can be selected as eliminating symptom.

5. USE OF CROSS-REPERTORIZATION

At times the case requires repertorization using 2 or 3 repertories which is termed as cross-repertorization. Cross repertorization requires different reportorial totalities to be made according to repertory used. When the rubrics in the reportorial totality are so selected that they are found in all the repertories used, it is termed as integrated cross repertorization; this is only possible if the case contains enough data which can be utilized from any angle. Cross repertorization is done to confirm the results obtained using one repertory. Similar results obtained using two repertories highlight the oneness of all repertories. Besides this, cross repertorization also considerably helps one to gain mastery over the process of repertorization as various repertories are used.

Repertorization brings together similar pictures and shows us the way to differentiate them. It furnishes the best possible systematic training in the evolution of patient's conceptual image as well as differential study of materia medica. A physician who frequently repertorises his cases would often find a progressive improvement in his case records which portray for him the indicated remedy unmistakably. It is seen that the physician who has mastered repertorization finds it least needed in his practice. Dr. M.L. Dhawale rightly states that, "A physician who has failed to grasp the fundamentals of repertorization fails to develop the right attitude to homeopathic practice and ends up as a mediocre prescriber."

Repertorization is a science based on the principles of inductive and deductive logic, generalization, & evaluation necessary in various operations of repertorization. It demands high degree of selectivity on part of the treating physician. We can conclude that scientific approach to repertorization consists of right selection of repertory before repertorization, acting in accordance with the philosophy of the repertory selected and application of the basic principles of repertorization, with correct interpretation of patient's expressions in reportorial terms. Last but not the least, having a logical base to the thought process during repertorization.

■

APPENDIX D

Format of Repertorial Syndrome

Patient's name:
Date: Case Index No:
Repertory Selected / Used:

Repertorial Syndrome / Totality

No.	Symptom	Rubric	Reason/Comment	Page No.
1.				
2.				
3.				
4.				
5.				
6.				
7.				
8.				
9.				
10.				

ILLUSTRATIVE CASE
(Perceiving Totality, Repertorial Syndrome and Remedy Differentiation)

Name: John Joseph (name changed)

Age: 10 years **Sex:** Male **Date:** February 10, 2005

Religion: Christian **Habit:** Non-veg **Occ.:** Student (6th standard)

Residential Address: 242 Samarth Nagar, Ajni, Nagpur, Pin – 440015

Referred by: Mr Vivek Mahajan

Father: Mr Anto Joseph **Age:** 38 years **Occ.:** Store incharge

Mother: Mrs Vaishali **Age:** 34 years **Occ.:** Staff nurse, Central Railways

Siblings: Brother 1 **Age:** 5 years **Occ.:** Student

PRESENT HISTORY

Chief Complaint

Location: Since 6 months of age (Respiratory Tract)

Sensation: Cough dry first and then turns wet, wheatish creamish thick expectoration, breathlessness, can't expectorate (would feel better if he could expectorate), rattling (> by Homeopathic treatment earlier but symptoms returned again since January 2003).

Modalities: Ailments from eating 'Shrikhand' in excess.

Aggravation from: Cold drinks^{2+}, sweets, January-February, talking, exertion, lying down, sitting^{2+}, winter^{2+}, rainy weather, fanning and draft of air.

Concomitants: Fever, averse to covers, weakness, thirst for small quantity, occasional throat pain.

Patient as a Person

Appearance: Blonde hair and eyebrows, brownish eyes with dark circles under eyes.

Height: 4ft.   **Weight**: 32kg.

Appetite: Eats thrice a day, 4 chappaties+ vegetables+ rice + dal.

Thirst: In 1 ½ – 2 hours, 1-2 glass at a time, likes cold water

Cravings: Chicken^{2+}, ghee^{2+}, fried–fish, pickles^{2+}, ice-cream^{2+}, sweets (peda), milk^{3+}, fried food^{3+} (Demands only parantha with excessive butter applied)

Aversion: Brinjal, vegetables^{2+}

Disagrees: Sweets (< cough), takes only peda

Stools: Passes stools once in 2 days, semi- solid stools offensive smelling

Urine: 7-8 times/day, no odours, no stains.

Sweat: Sweats all over the body (< exertion), more on face and back. No stains, no odour.

Life Space

Mother's version: Quiet nature, talks and plays with those whom he likes. He does not do the work completely which has been told by his mother. Likes maths, studies on his own. Does not like to talk to girls of any age and does not want a sister also. Gets angry a lot when he is right and anybody tells that no he is wrong, but does not express his anger and cries. Likes play more than to study. He feels that his friends should not go to anybody else. He feels that he should stand first in academics; he tries a lot but no considerable change in rank, feels depressed and weeps if somebody says he can't do anything.

He does not like if somebody teases his brother. His father, most of the times stay out of station for weeks or days. He misses his father on special occasions. Fear of mother makes him sit for studies otherwise in her absence he is only interested in maths. He has fear of dark, gets frightened easily.

He wants to be a doctor or a pilot. At night can't go to the toilet alone. Father is from Christian family and mother from Hindu. He did not want any siblings and got angry after his brother was born, as he has to share things whereas his friends are the only child and get many things which do not have to be shared. Does not weep in front of someone, will go to toilet and weep easily. He doesn't like his mother to be around as she asks him to study. He is lazy when it comes to study. Averse to any household job.

First child in Joseph family and was pampered by all. Breast fed for 4 ½ years, was difficult to wean.

He was frightened by telling that the policeman will hit him and put him in jail if he did not give up breast feeding.

Sleep and Dreams: Wants to sleep more (10 pm – 6 am). He dreams of flying aircraft, being awarded for playing cricket, flying kite, playing games. Talks in sleep.

Physical Reactions

Bathing: Throughout the season with warm water

Covering: Averse to covers[2+], does not like to cover in summer, only if it is cool then takes blanket

Food: Likes warm food

Season: Likes summer

Fanning: Likes fanning < cough, winter < cough

In summers, nose bleeds (since 2-3years) only when exposed to sun for 3-4 hours.

Family History

Paternal Grandfather: High blood pressure, MGF- admitted in hospital and expired

Paternal Grandmother: High blood pressure

Father: Migraine

Past History

Chicken pox: 7 years of age

Head injury from falling from a wall when 1 ½ years old

Hospitalised 2-3 times at the age of 2-4years of age for complaint of cough

Weight gain from 3 months to 5-6years

Nose bleeding in summer season

Bedwetting since one year

Gestational notes

- Had craving for mud
- FTND
- Didn't want the child and had gone for abortion but relative told to keep so she did
- Used to think that she has conceived early and it was an early responsibility

- Episiotomy had been given
- Birth weight: 1.65 kg.
- Lactation: till 4 ½ yrs.
- Lochia: for one month

Milestones

Head holding: 3 months

Sitting with support: 6-7 months

Sitting without support: 8-9 months

Crawling: Used to take support of one leg

Monosyllables: 10 months

Speech: 1 year 9 months

Standing: 10 months

Walking: 11 months

Dentition: 7 months (had loose motion, used to pass frequently)

Pica: No

Vaccinations: All vaccinations given

Physical Findings

Pallor: Absent

Icterus: Absent

Pulse: 90/ min.

Tongue: Clear and moist

Cardiovascular System: NAD

Gastrointestinal System: NAD

Other findings
- Scar on head
- Macular eruption on right middle finger

CASE PROCESSING

Diagnosis: Chronic Bronchitis

Features in favour

1. Cough, which is initially dry then becomes wet with creamish thick expectoration.
2. Breathlessness and difficulty in expectoration accompanied by fever and rattling in chest.
3. Aggravation of the complaints in winter (Jan – Feb) and aggravation in rainy weather (these are aggravating factors in bronchitis giving rise to acute exacerbations).

TOTALITY OF SYMPTOMS

Family History
- High blood pressure
- Migraine

Past History
- Chicken pox
- Head injury
- Obese

Mental State

Intellect: Mediocre

Emotion: Fear, demanding, obstinate

Behaviour: Possessive, timid

Functioning: Indolent

Thermality: Chilly

Generals: <Winter^{2+}, cold Drinks^{2+}, drafts^{2+}, covers^{2+}, talking^{2+}, fanning >Warm drink^{2+}, sitting^{2+}

Mental: Irritable^{2+}, anger, fear^{2+} of darkness, sadness, weeping^{2+}, jealousy

Dreams: Pleasent^{2+}, fanciful, talking in sleep

Craving: Fats^{2+}, chicken^{2+}, ice-creams^{2+}, milk^{3+}

Aversion: Vegetables^{2+}, sweets^{+}

CHARACTERISTIC PARTICULARS

- < Winter^{2+}, cold drinks^{2+}, drafts^{2+}, talking^{2+}, fanning
- >Warm drink^{2+}, sitting^{2+}
- Cough
- Difficult, thick, creamish expectoration
- Breathlessness
- Respiratory tract
- Stools: constipated, offensive^{+}
- Rectum

REPERTORIAL SYNDROME

Repertory Used: BTPB (Boenninghausen's Therapeutic Pocket Book)

SYMPTOM	RUBRIC	COMMENT	PAGE NO.
<Winter^{2+}	<Winter, in	Physical General	310
<Cold Drinks^{2+}	<Food and drink, cold	Physical General	282
<Drafts^{2+}	<Draft	Physical General	277
<Covers^{2+}	<Warm wraps	Physical General	308
<Talking^{2+}	<Talking	Physical General	303
>Sitting^{2+}	>Sitting	Important Modality	319
Susceptible to cold	Cold tendency to take	Physical General	148
Irritable^{2+}	Irritability	Mental General	18

Emerging Chronic Chilly Remedies

- Calc. carb – 28/8
- Sil. – 26/7
- Sepia – 25/7
- Caust. – 19/7
- Ferr – 19/6
- Nit.ac. – 18/6
- Kali c. – 17/6
- Phos – 16/7
- Bar. carb – 16/6
- Petr – 16/5
- Con – 15/5
- Graph – 14/5
- Aur – 14/4

Scientific Approach to Repertorization

POTENTIAL DIFFERENTIAL FIELD

Repertory Used: Kent's Repertory

SYMPTOM	RUBRIC	COMMENT	PAGE NO.
Obstinate	Mind	Obstinate	69
Timid	Mind	Timidity	88
Fear of darkness	Mind	Fear dark	43
Indolent	Mind	Indolence, Aversion to work	55
Weeping	Mind	Weeping, tearful mood	92
Craving : Fats[2+]	Stomach	Desires, Fat	485
Craving : Milk[3+]	Stomach	Desires, Milk	485
Aversion : Vegetables[2+]	Stomach	Aversion, Vegetables	482

Emerging Remedies

- Calc. carb. - 15/6
- Phos - 10/5

DIFFERENTIATION OF EMERGING REMEDIES

Differentiation - Mental level: The patient is demanding, obstinate and fearful. He is possessive, timid and indolent, having aversion to household work and lazy about studies. He has a mediocre intellect. This mental state makes him irritable, weepy and jealous. He is having fear of darkness.

First drug for consideration is Calcarea carbonica. Patient's mind comes closer to Calcarea carbonica and the drug covers the obstinacy, demanding nature and fearfulness. Like the patient Calcarea carbonica is also inactive or indolent having aversion to mental as well as physical work. Also the obstinacy and the fact that he is indolent results in failure and this makes him irritable. In both the patient and Calcarea carbonica we get the expressions of anger, sadness, weeping fear of dark and jealousy. Thus, patient's mind can be seen in Calcarea carbonica.

If we compare Phosphorus, we see that it also has fear, sadness, irritability, jealousy and weeping but patient's mind differs from that of Phosphorus. The patient is indolent and inactive while Phosphorus individual is active. Patient is demanding and obstinate while Phosphorus is weak-willed and escapist, although both are timid. Patient is intellectually a mediocre whereas Phosphorus is intellectually keen. In the patient the indolence is giving rise to failure and is responsible for irritability and sadness, while in Phosphorus irritability and sadness arise due to the weak will and keen intellect giving rise to erratic activity and thereby to failure. Thus, patient differs a lot from Phosphorus at mental level.

Differentiation –Physical generals: This patient is chilly, aggravated by winter^{2+}, cold drinks^{2+}, drafts^{2+}, covers^{2+}, talking^{2+} and fanning; ameliorated by warm drinks^{2+} and sitting^{2+}. Has craving for fried^{3+}, fats^{2+}, chicken, ice-cream^{2+} and milk^{3+}. Aversion to vegetables^{2+}. He is having pleasent^{2+} and fanciful dreams, talks in sleep and has sweats^{+}.

Calcarea carbonica is a chilly drug and covers <winter, drafts, covers, talking and fanning. It also covers > sitting and warm drinks. Calcarea carbonica has craving for cold drinks, ice-creams, fats and fried, but craving for chicken is not seen. Calcarea carbonica has aversion to milk. The aversion for vegetables is not covered by Calcarea carbonica. It covers pleasant and fanciful dreams and talking in sleep and also the sweats^{+}.

Phosphorus covers < drafts, cold drinks and fanning whereas <winter is not marked in Phosphorus. The <talking is covered by Phosphorus. The contradictory thing about modalities is that Phosphorus has aversion to uncovering and wants covers and has <sitting. Craving for fried fats and chicken is not covered by Phosphorus. Phosphorus has aversion to milk especially boiled milk; also the aversion to vegetables is not covered by Phosphorus. Phosphorus only covers craving for ice-creams. Phosphorus also covers talking in sleep but does not cover pleasant and fanciful dreams. It covers the sweats[+]. Thus, Phosphorus falls back in general modalities and cravings and aversions, it is therefore less close to patient's physical generals. Calcarea carbonica stands better in case of physical generals.

Differentiation - Characteristic particulars: Characteristic particulars of the patient are

- Cough with thick, creamish expectoration and breathlessness
- <winter^{2+}, cold drinks^{2+}, drafts^{2+}, talking^{2+} and fanning
- \> warm drinks^{2+} and sitting^{2+}
- Constipated and offensive stools

Calcarea carbonica covers cough, breathlessness with thick creamish expectoration, < winter, drafts, talking^{2+} and fanning and >sitting and warm drinks. It also covers < cold drinks.

It also covers constipated and offensive stools but has hard stools evacuated with difficulty which is characteristic at particular level. Calcarea carbonica thus covers the patient's characteristic particulars. Phoshorus covers cough and breathlessness, < cold drinks, talking, drafts and fanning but thick creamish expectoration is not covered by Phoshorus. It has bloody and rust-coloured expectoration which is marked. It also doesn't cover the accompanying modalities of >warm drinks and sitting. It covers the constipated and offensive stool but in Phoshorus the diarrohoea is more prominent then constipation.

REMEDY SELECTION

After comparing these drugs at the level of mind, physical generals and characteristic particulars patient's image comes close to the remedy Calcarea carbonica at all the three levels and it is therefore the simillimum for the patient.

∎

CHAPTER 10

Working Methods of Repertorization

- ❖ Methods in General   227
- ❖ Methods According to Philosophical Background   232

CHAPTER 10

WORKING METHODS OF REPERTORIZATION

A physician must have complete knowledge of the particular repertory he wishes to use. Besides, knowledge regarding the various methods of repertorization is equally essential for repertorization to be scientific.

Method of Repertorization means the process by which repertorization is carried out. The word 'method' is used to indicate the actual procedure carried out on paper, using tabulations in different styles. It also denotes the way in which repertorial totality is constructed for repertorization. Here method means style of working based on the philosophy of the repertory one is using. Every repertory differs in its construction and philosophy from the others. Methods have evolved from the philosophy underlying each repertory.

METHODS IN GENERAL

Methods depending on the actual process carried out for repertorization are as follows:

1. Thumb-finger Method or Fingering Process.
2. Old Method or Plain Paper Method.
3. Modern Method or Repertorial Sheet Method.
4. Mechanical Method (Cards, Computer and Auto-visual).
5. Eliminating Method.
6. Total Addition Process.

1. THUMB-FINGER METHOD

Sheet of paper or tabulations are not used in this method. It is a time saving method meant for quick reference. This method is only suitable for physician's having a good experience of using repertories. Neophytes should avoid using this method, as errors are inevitable in this method if one is not careful. In thumb-finger method the physician only refers to required rubrics having in mind few probable remedies for the case. Usually two or three characteristics are taken and the repertory is searched. While searching the physician places the thumb and fingers between pages and compares different rubrics. Thus he arrives at 2 to 3 probable remedies out of which one would be prescribed after consulting materia medica. This method is useful in a busy practice.

However, errors are inevitable if the number of medicines listed against the rubrics are too many.

2. OLD METHOD OR PLAIN PAPER METHOD

It is the most time consuming and laborious method. It is known as old method due to the fact that it was used in the early years when the repertories had just arrived and tabulated sheets were yet to be discovered. In this method rubrics are arranged according to their order of importance and medicines are listed against them on a plain paper. All medicines with their grades are written by hand against the symptoms. At the end common medicines covering all the rubrics are found out. They are further differentiated using materia medica to arrive at the prescription.

The advantage of this method is that while referring to the rubrics and noting down the medicines with grades one gets well acquainted with the repertory, as it leaves a lasting impression on the user's memory. Thus, it proves useful in improving the knowledge of repertory as well as materia medica.

3. MODERN METHOD OR REPERTORIAL SHEET METHOD

It is a better and time saving method as compared to the old method. In this method tabulated sheet is used. This tabulated repertorial sheet contains an alphabetically arranged list of medicines on left hand side and sufficient number of columns to record grades of medicines in front of them. Marks are given in the columns against each medicine, according to its value mentioned in the repertory.

The disadvantage of this method is that the difference between rubrics covered and marks obtained by leading remedies may lead to confusion.

4. MECHANICAL METHOD

This includes use of cards, computer and auto-visual apparatus for repertorization.

(a) Card Method

Card repertories are actually devices that help in rapid repertorization. Card repertories consist of set of cards. The rubrics are printed on the top of cards. The remedies covering the rubric are listed below and punched. Different types of punches are used for indicating the gradation. Size of the card differs with each card repertory.

Card repertories are suitable for busy practitioners as they cut down the time needed in calculation and paper work is not required. The disadvantages are blocking of remedies, and difficulty in calculating marks due to lack of gradation of remedies. Sometimes the rubric selected is not found, as card repertories contain limited no of rubrics. Handling is difficult if the total number of cards is more. There is a chance of cards getting torn or destroyed over a period of time due to ageing of card paper.

(b) Computer Aided Method

Card repertories have taken a back stage since the arrival of computers, as they are more refined devices containing more number of rubrics as compared to card repertories. Computers are electronic devices used for repertorization. A case is repertorized in the shortest time once the rubrics are selected. Computer repertories have revolutionized the process of repertorization. The searching of rubrics, comparison with other repertories, reference to materia medica and cross-repertorization has become easy as everything is available on screen just at the press of a button. It is advantageous but the advantages depend on the type of software programme one is using. One must not forget that a computer cannot replace a reason gifted human mind. Computer only gives back what is fed to it. RADAR, which has been developed in Belgium, is considered the most comprehensive and easy-to-use software.

(c) Auto-visual Repertory

It is a mechanical device of repertorization developed by Dr. R. P. Patel of Kerala, India. No paperwork is required. It is automatic and only 10 to 15 minutes are required to repertorize a case once the rubrics are selected. It consists of 5505 autostrips. This apparatus is based on Kent's Repertory and contains 435 remedies. Each medicine is provided with a code number. Every autostrip is grooved at several places. Each groove on the autostrip represents corresponding homeopathic medicine. The grooves are in different colours or markings to indicate gradation of remedies.

Drugs of highest value shown in capitals in Kent's repertory are coloured red in auto-visual apparatus. It indicates numerical value 3. The drugs in italics in Kent's repertory are coloured yellow and have numerical value 2, while drugs in plain or roman type in Kent's repertory are coloured black and have numerical value 1. Again, there are two heavy grooves (Green), one at the top and one at the bottom of the autostrips as "Guidelines." Autostrip numbers are also coloured, some are red and some are black. This is to indicate the type of symptom. General symptoms are coloured in red and particulars in black. This helps in selecting the symptoms and placing the autostrips in the auto-visual apparatus in the order of importance i.e. mentals, physical generals and particulars. The autostrips are fed in auto-visual apparatus. The apparatus has space for 10 autostrips. A single straight horizontal line is obtained after feeding the selected autostrips. If more than one horizontal line is obtained, these are competing remedies which match all the rubics.

5. ELIMINATING METHOD

The eliminating method was introduced by Margaret Tyler and Sir John Weir. They advocated the use of this method to cut short the repertory work. In the eliminating method while constructing the repertorial totality the most important and characteristic symptom of the patient without which the prescription cannot be thought of is selected as an eliminating symptom. This symptom is placed on the top and the rest of the symptoms are placed below it according to hierarchy. Only those medicines which cover the first symptom or the eliminating symptom are taken while repertorizing. Further rubrics can be referred to and marks added to only those medicines that are covered by eliminating symptom.

This method narrows down the list of emerging remedies. Eliminating method is time saving, less confusing and easy to practice if followed properly. It cuts the labour without compromising the quality of repertorization. Some physicians are of the opinion that up to 2 or 3 symptoms can be taken as eliminating symptoms. This reduces the chances of loosing the indicated remedy in the eliminating process. This is known as *continuous elimination.* Rubrics having one or few remedies should not be taken as eliminating rubrics.

Generals, important concomitants and pathological generals in cases with advanced pathology can be taken as eliminating rubrics.

6. TOTAL ADDITION PROCESS

In total addition process all medicines against all rubrics are noted down and finally total marks scored by each remedy are calculated. Medicines having higher marks are further differentiated. In this method possibility of omitting a remedy is less. Both old as well as the modern method can be used while working with this process. It is suitable to Kent, Boenninghausen as well as Boger's repertory. The only disadvantage is that it is a time consuming process.

METHODS ACCORDING TO PHILOSOPHICAL BACKGROUND

Methods of repertorization according to philosophical background of repertories are as follows:

1. Hahnemann and Boenninghausen's Method.
2. Kent's Method.
3. Working on Physical Generals.
4. Working on Peculiarity.
5. Working on Pathological Changes.
6. Working on Technical Nosology.

1. HAHNEMANN AND BOENNINGHAUSEN'S METHOD

This method is useful in cases where complete symptoms are available. It is especially useful in cases where mental generals are deficient and particular symptoms and concomitants are more prominently present. This method is useful while repertorizing cases with Boenninghausen's Therapeutic Pocket Book. In this method locations, sensations, modalities and concomitants are taken as rubrics. The disadvantage of this method is that the list of rubrics become larger and physician has to refer large rubrics, hence it makes repertorization time consuming and laborious. This method is also known as Robert's method.

2. KENT'S METHOD

It is suitable for well taken cases where both the generals as well as particulars are available. In this method important generals and particulars are taken for repertorization. Mental symptoms are placed at the top. This method is most suitable for working with Kent's philosophy. It is the most commonly used method.

3. WORKING ON PHYSICAL GENERALS

It is suitable where mental generals are deficient. In this method physical generals are taken first followed by mentals. It is suitable for working with Boenninghausen Therapeutic Pocket Book and Kent's repertory.

4. WORKING ON PECULIARITY

In this method striking and peculiar symptoms are used for repertorization. It is especially suitable where case is deficient in well-defined symptoms and generals.

5. WORKING ON PATHOLOGICAL CHANGES

This method should be used in cases where only pathology and common symptoms are available and the physician is expected to prescribe on these alone. In such cases physician has to use every means available at his disposal. Here following features can prove useful:

(i) Patient's personal and family history.
(ii) Temperament.
(iii) Complexion, colour and texture of skin.
(iv) Particular organs and tissues affected.
(v) Location, character and physical aspect of lesions.
(vi) Probable etiological factors.

6. WORKING ON TECHNICAL NOSOLOGY

Here technical nosological terms are selected as main headings. It is suitable for working with clinical repertories like Boericke's repertory. This method should be only resorted to when nothing else is available, because use of nosological terms for selection of medicine is contrary to homeopathic teachings and most of the time ends in failure. The chances of finding the right remedy are greatly reduced by concentrating on nosological diagnosis. A secondary importance should be given to nosological labels while selecting the remedy. Searching the *simillimum* for totality of symptoms is the right way and in accordance with homeopathic principles. Only this proves useful in the long run.

All methods have their advantages and disadvantages and, therefore, it is better to use the method that is best for the case in question. Only by following the homeopathic teachings of giving prime importance to the characteristic symptoms one can do justice to his patients.

■

CHAPTER 11

How to Select the Right Remedy ?

- ❖ Right Thinking for Right Selection — 240
- ❖ Establishing Similarity — 243
- ❖ Criteria for Establishing Similarity — 245
- ❖ Self-Assessment — 246
- ❖ Techniques of Prescribing — 247
- ❖ Inference — 253

CHAPTER 11

HOW TO SELECT THE RIGHT REMEDY?

What allopathy means by an indicated remedy is quiet different from what homeopaths call a homeopathically suitable remedy. Every homeopath knows this but still it needs to be mentioned here, because very few amongst us follow the principles, logic and the rules governing remedy selection in actual practice. According to Hahnemann there are three errors that we are all liable to make, "1st the selection of improper remedy, 2nd the improper potency and 3rd not letting the remedy act a sufficient length of time."

Majority of present day homeopaths employ erroneous methods of remedy selection. Some try to search for specific and rare remedies for a particular disease condition. They prescribe for the 'disease' and not for the 'patient.' Some use a particular remedy just because they have heard of its effectiveness in XYZ disease. Hahnemann describes the third type of homeopaths who heavily rely on repertory for remedy selection. He states that, *"A man who thus is satisfied with the vague hints of repertory in the selection of a remedy and quickly gets through with one patient after the other, is rather a quack, and will then have to give a new remedy every minute, until the patient loses his patience, and his ailments having been, as may easily be understood, aggravated he leaves such an aggravator of disease who throws discredit on the art instead of merely the unworthy disciple of this art."*

Prescribing a remedy because of its high score in repertorization, prescribing on pathology, prescribing on laboratory investigation and other such methods of remedy selection are unscientific methods of remedy selection. These methods are unreliable because they are unhomeopathic. A homeopath who employs these methods is bound to fail in majority of cases. This miserable picture has emerged from the fact that academicians and those involved in training of a homeopath pay very little attention to teaching the right methods of remedy selection. There is an increasing tendency to neglect homeopathic philosophy and logic amongst practitioners. A fresh homeopathic graduate therefore often gets confused due to the whims and notions of various schools that have emerged in homeopathy in the recent years. He has no clear-cut ideas regarding the logical methods and techniques of remedy selection. Therefore, it is necessary to address the question of remedy selection in the light of homeopathic philosophy and logic.

Let us see. After the totality is made and the case repertorized, the physician proceeds to find out the remedy that resembles patient's totality to the maximum. The 'selection' like all other operations in homeopathic practice, is governed by the principle of individualization. Perhaps this is what makes it most difficult and crucial operation in homeopathic practice especially made more difficult when the case is complicated one. The real test of efficiency of a genuine homeopath lies in his ability to select the right remedial agent for curing. Everyone agrees that correct choice of remedy is a difficult task. The obvious question that arises from this fact is, what a homeopathician is expected to do while selecting the remedy for his patient? This question, has a better answer if we understand what one should not do while selecting the remedy. Where to find the answer to this important question? The answer is simple. Hahnemann's 'Organon' which is in fact Hahnemann's guide to homeopathic practice, contains the guidelines which primarily deal with the 'thought process' required and the precautions that need to be taken while selecting the simillimum. He has dealt with these guidelines in paragraphs 18, 153, 257 and 258 of Organon of Medicine. If carefully interpreted one realizes that through these aphorisms Hahnemann has actually elaborated on the prejudiced thinking habits a physician should guard against while selecting a suitable remedy.

Hahnemann clearly states in aphorism 18 that totality is the only indication and only guide to selection of remedy.

> "From this indubitable truth, that besides the totality of the symptoms, with consideration of the accompanying modalities nothing can by any means be discovered in diseases wherewith they could express their need of aid, it follows undeniably that the sum of all the symptoms and conditions in each individual case of disease must be the sole indication, the sole guide to direct us in the choice of a remedy."
>
> **— Samuel Hahnemann**
> (Paragraph 18 of Organon of Medicine)

It won't be wrong to call any prescription as unhomeopathic if it falls out of this basic rule given by Hahnemann. Some may call it 'classical homeopathy.' But these divisions of homeopathy are made by us. Hahnemann never thought of various types of homeopathy or prescribing. He knew that the basic law on which his science is based is law of similars and hence, he clearly stated that totality is the soul guide to homeopathic prescription and nothing else.

Prescribing remedy on the basis of reportorial result (one which scores highest marks), prescribing on diagnostic symptoms, pathology or laboratory investigations and other such methods of drug selection are unhomeopathic methods of prescription making and therefore not advisable, except in cases with paucity of symptoms. Kent in his lectures on homeopathic philosophy says that, "The more you dwell upon diagnostic symptoms, the more you becloud the ideas entering the mind that lead towards prescription." Kent thus describes in a single sentence the crux of the type of thought process necessary for homeopathic prescription making.

RIGHT THINKING FOR RIGHT SELECTION

Correct choice of remedy largely depends on the thought process carried out in the mind of the physician at the time of prescribing. Only if the way of thinking is 'homeopathic' enough, one can have repeated success in remedy selection. Homeopathic thinking means thinking free of prejudice and in accordance with the principles and logic of homeopathy. Blocks in thinking are primarily responsible for errors in selection. Right thinking results from right approach to prescribing. It is the soul of a good prescription. Apart from absence of prejudices the ability to differentiate remedy portraits, mastery over the art of perceiving totality while matching patient's image to drug image are other essential prerequisites necessary for the clinical thinking to be truly 'homeopathic.'

It needs to be clearly understood what constitutes 'unprejudiced clinical thinking' which is must for correct choice of remedy. We find the answer to this in paragraphs 153, 257 & 258 of Organon of Medicine.

> "The true physician will take care to avoid making favorite remedies of medicines, the employment of which he has, by chance, perhaps found often useful, and which he has had opportunities of using with good effect. If he do so, some remedies of rarer use, which

would have been more homeopathically suitable, consequently more serviceable, will often be neglected."

— **Samuel Hahnemann**
(Paragraph 257 of Organon)

"The true practitioner, moreover, will not in his practice with mistrustful weakness neglect the employment of those remedies that he may now and then have employed with bad effects, owing to an erroneous selection (from his own fault, therefore), or avoid them for other (false) reasons, as that they were unhomeopathic for the case of disease before him; he must bear in mind the truth, that of medicinal agents that one alone invariably deserves the preference in every case of disease which corresponds most accurately by similarity to the totality of the characteristic symptoms, and that no paltry prejudices should interfere with this serious choice."

— **Samuel Hahnemann**
(Paragraph 258 of Organon)

In aphorism 153, Hahnemann has tried to explain what is meant by total correspondence of patient's symptoms to drug symptoms. He has advised the physician to concentrate on more striking, singular, uncommon and peculiar signs and symptoms of the case. He states that the selected medicine can be called a true simillimum only if it corresponds to these (characteristic) symptoms of the patient. From his statements we can conclude that total correspondence means correspondence of characteristics or of essential attributes of the case with those of remedy selected. Total correspondence is therefore a qualitative concept, which involves matching of qualities of the two (i.e. patient's totality and drug totality) and not the quantity. This brings us to the fact that a physician is expected to concentrate on characteristics while prescribing. This is the first step towards 'homeopathic' selection of the curing agent.

Hahnemann was well aware of the pitfalls of homeopathic prescribing. He fully knew what might go wrong while selecting a drug, and hence in paragraph 257 of Organon of Medicine, he warns the physician to avoid employment of 'favourite remedies.' The favourite remedies are those which have been repeatedly employed with good results by a physician. Every successful application of a certain remedy improves a physician's grasp over its curing capabilities but paradoxically it also makes the remedy his favourite and this usually results in its overuse. It is very natural for a physician to think of one or two such favourites while searching for simillimum. But by routinely prescribing the favourites, physician neglects other drugs which might have proved more similar to the case in hand. Consciously avoiding the thinking of favourite remedies, which is a natural tendency, is another important part of what constitutes unprejudiced clinical thinking.

Another erroneous way of prescribing to be avoided is prescribing a remedy just because 'you have heard that' it gives great results in a particular disease. Hahnemann warns against this erroneous practice in the footnote to paragraph 285 of Organon by stating that, "To prescribe for the sick on mere conjecture of some possible usefulness for some similar disease or from hearsay that a remedy has helped in such and such a disease, such conscienceless venture the philanthropic homeopathist will leave to the allopath."

FAULTY (PREJUDICED) THOUGHT PROCESS
Selecting a remedy because:
- It is a favourite remedy.
- It matches the pathological condition.
- It has scored highest in repertorization.
- It is used by other homeopaths with good results for a particular disease condition.
- It has given good results earlier.
- It matches the disease symptoms.
- It is full of symptoms belonging to system or organs involved in the case.

Similarly another pitfall of homeopathic prescription making is avoiding the use of some drugs, which have been employed with bad results repeatedly. Hahnemann calls this a 'mistrustful weakness' and a 'paltry prejudice' in paragraph 258 of Organon of Medicine. It must not be forgotten that if certain remedy has proved failure, it is not because the remedy didn't have the ability to give results. It was an erroneous selection and therefore bound to fail. Labelling some drugs as black sheep and avoiding their use is thus also a type of faulty clinical thinking, which a physician must not fall prey to. Only the drug that bears total correspondence to the patient's totality must be preferred without beclouding one's thoughts by earlier experiences with that particular drug which might have been good or bad.

ESTABLISHING SIMILARITY

What does the term 'similar' means must be understood very well before trying to establish similarity between natural disease and artificial disease. If a physician clearly understands the meaning by the term similar then only he is in a position to keep the mental process carried out for remedy selection on right lines.

According to English dictionary 'similar' means like, of same sort, resembling or in geometric terms corresponding in shape without regard to size, or similar means nearly equal in any respect but not exactly same. We should note here that similarity does not mean 'exact sameness.' When we say he looks like a particular actor, we do not mean that he is the exact copy of the film actor or identical to the actor, but we mean that his appearance has similar qualities (features) as that of the said actor. Following example will make it very clear.

When I say that 'this sweater is similar to the one I purchased last year' it means it is of similar sort or similar kind to the one purchased last year but does not mean it is absolutely same as the one purchased last year. Thus when two things are compared and it is stated that the two things are identical it means we are mentioning their exact sameness but it is different when it is stated that the two things are similar as it means that they resemble each other but are not exact replicas of each other. Dr. K. N. Kasad explains this very well in his paper on repertorization when he states that, "Similarity is an approximation to identity and not the same thing as identity. The concept of identity is the quality or condition of absolute or essential sameness or of oneness. It implies sharing all the attributes, traits, qualities and characteristics of an object or a phenomenon by another in its totality of form, function and structure." He further elaborates, "The concept of similarity is the condition or state of likeness, resemblance, correspondence between the two not absolute identity." Thus, we can conclude that what is identical can be similar but what is similar cannot be identical.

Similarly while we are searching for a similar remedy we are not searching for exact sameness but we want a remedial agent that resembles patient's portrait in terms of characteristic features. We are actually searching for a drug having similar qualities but not exactly same as the patient. This means that we would not find all the symptoms of the patient in the drug neither we would find all the symptoms of the drug in the patient. There would be some qualities which would not be shared by the two. The 'symptom pattern' of the patient should correspond to that of a drug and not all the symptoms. Thus establishing similarity cannot be done by matching all the symptoms or matching the numerical totality; it is different. It is necessary to keep in mind that Hahnemann expects a clinician to establish similarity not at the level of signs and symptoms but at the level of 'portrait,' because homeopathic specific is actually individual specific and not the disease specific. Hahnemann states this in Para. 154 of Organon of Medicine.

Error in establishing similarity often results from attempting to fit a remedy to a patient. It is the most faulty method of establishing similarity. Physician's aim should always be to see whether the patient fits a certain remedy or not. He should proceed from patient to the remedy and never in the reverse order while comparing.

CRITERIA FOR ESTABLISHING SIMILARITY

Knowing what similarity means does not guarantee success in selection of the right remedy. Besides, the physician ought to know the various aspects of similarity that need to be considered while establishing similarity. Following points can serve as the essential parameters for establishing similarity while matching the patient's totality to the drug totality.

1. Matching of 'portrait' of the patient and the remedy which includes consideration of symptom patterns or patient's image rather than patient's symptoms. Matching of images or portraits which means that symptoms should not be considered separately but the manner in which they are grouped together has to be studied while comparing.

2. Matching the characteristic symptomatic expressions at the three levels i.e. mental level, level of physical generals and at the level of particulars. Besides this, it is also essential to consider functional and structural level of disease evolution.

3. Matching the type or phase of disease expression in the patient to that in a particular drug's symptomatology. This takes into consideration the type of presentation — acute, chronic, periodic appearance of symptoms, cyclic, alternating and relapsing states.

4. Establishing similarity at both the central as well as peripheral level of expressions is important. Central similarity is the

similarity of the core of the patient's image. Core consists of commanding features of the case at both the mental and physical level and the constitutional peculiarities i.e. diathesis, temperament, and causative factors, etc. By peripheral expressions is meant the symptoms at the level of particulars. Peripheral similarity can only lead to suppression of symptoms and never a cure. Many drugs have almost same or very similar peripheral expressions but they differ at the central level.

5. Establishing close similarity should be the physician's prime aim and only partial similarity can never cure the patient hence the degree of similarity also needs consideration. A partial similarity can only alter patient's symptom picture making the case more difficult for treatment. But only in case of one-sided diseases where remedy having total similarity cannot be selected due to paucity of symptoms, Hahnemann advises us to administer partially similar remedial agent. He further states that after prescribing this partial simillimum some symptoms become more perceptible and the whole collection of symptoms i.e. those present before the prescription and those that have appeared after its administration, have to be considered and a new remedy needs to be selected on the basis of this picture that presents itself after the first prescription. These guidelines we find in paragraphs from 179 to paragraph 184 of Organon of Medicine.

6. Matching not only the portraits but also the potency, dose and repetition according to patients susceptibility and the demands of the case, so that the drug selected is complete simillimum or potential simillimum.

SELF-ASSESSMENT

Examining one's own thinking pattern while selecting a remedy must be done from time to time to reduce faulty prescribing habits to the minimum. For this one needs to ask oneself certain questions. This self-assessment is a sure way of knowing exactly where one may go wrong while prescribing as it automatically reveals the truth about our faulty thinking habits which serve as a major obstacle in correct prescribing. The self-assessment questions can be listed as follows:

1. Do I acquire all the data necessary for making homeopathic prescription? When it is not available do I try to prescribe on the type of pathology, part affected or other signs of disease or I make efforts to get what is needed for correct choice?
2. Are there any remedies that I frequently prescribe? If yes do I consider them very effective as compared to others consciously or unconsciously ?
3. Are there any remedies that I seldom prescribe, because perhaps I know very little about them?
4. Do I differentiate between common and uncommon symptoms of the patient before I select a suitable remedy?
5. What is my understanding of the concept of totality? Is it in accordance with the one laid down by Hahnemann? Do I fully understand the practical implications of the concept also?
6. While searching for simillimum, am I in the habit of directly going to materia medica to see if the symptoms of a particular drug resemble the patient's symptoms? or I do the reverse i.e. thorough study the case in the first place to assess the totality and then going to materia medica.

TECHNIQUES OF PRESCRIBING

Technique can be defined as that part of art that can be reduced to formula. Homeopathy by virtue of its principle of individualization cannot be made to fit into any formula or fixed technique. Similar is the case with the homeopathic prescription. It varies with the patient and the circumstances present at the time of prescribing. However, with accumulation of clinical experience certain techniques develop automatically. It is a slow process and it happens when a discriminating physician applies the principles

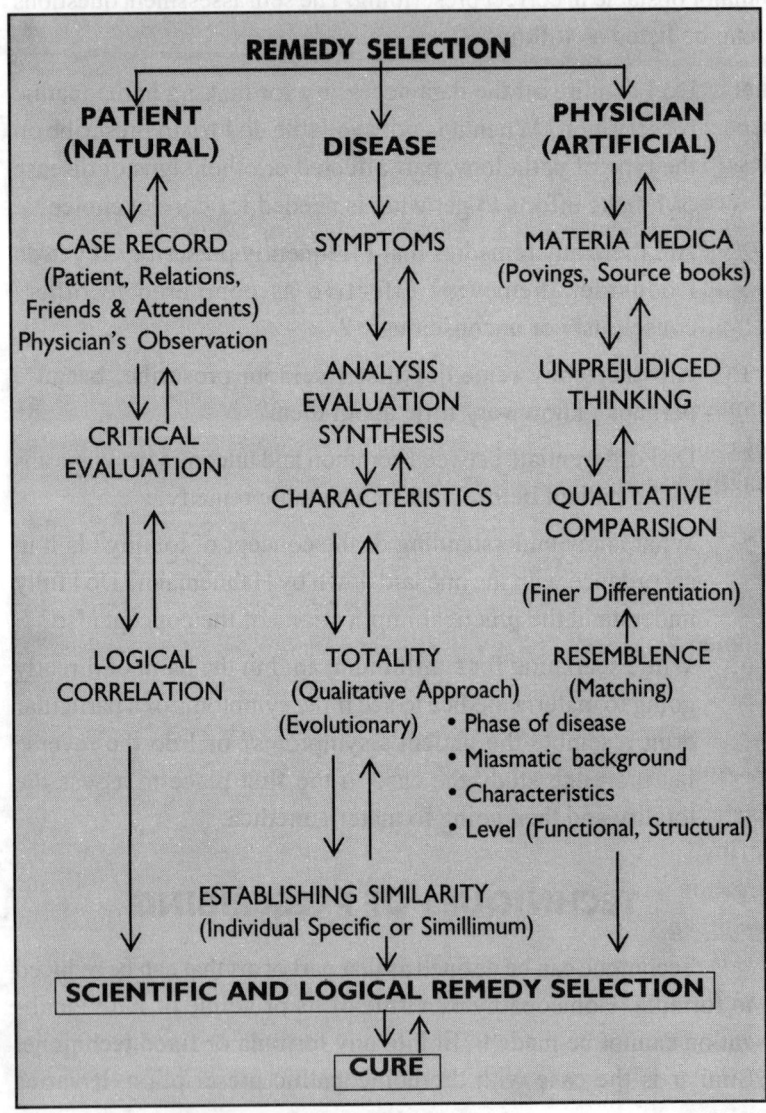

in his practice for considerable period of time. The present era homeopaths are fortunate that various homeopathic stalwarts through their hard work and exigencies of their practice have evolved certain methods of prescribing without departing from the law in the process.

The nature of the case in hand decides the aspects of totality that need to be considered while prescribing. The techniques have been developed keeping in mind this point of view. The techniques described here will give the reader a general frame of reference that can be used while prescribing.

Hahnemann broadly classified the diseases into acute and chronic. This classification permits clear-cut understanding of disease expression. Acute and chronic diseases are not separate entities. They are the two phases of a continuous spectrum of deranged vitality. The techniques, therefore, also need to be grouped into acute and chronic prescribing. The method of prescription making varies with the phase of disease expression.

I. ACUTE PRESCRIBING

Acute diseases have rapid course and are usually self-limiting. The acute diseases may supervene in the course of the chronic diseases due to the adverse environmental factors.

There is a general tendency amongst homeopaths to look for specifics in acute conditions, but the simillimum indicated at that particular moment is the only known specific. Hahnemann has defined the term homeopathic specific in paragraph 154 of Organon. He states, " *If the antitype constructed from the list of symptoms of the most suitable medicine contain those peculiar, uncommon, singular and distinguishing (characteristic) symptoms, which are to be met within the disease to be cured in the greatest number and in the greatest similarity, this medicine is the most appropriate homeopathic specific remedy.*" To find out this specific, the presenting totality consisting of chief complaint and concomitants is taken into consideration. The characteristic location, sensations, modalities and concomitants govern the remedy selection in acute cases. The differentiating modalities are a sure guide to the remedy. The characteristic modalities, for example time modalities (*Ars.* midday midnight aggravation, *Lyco., Coloc.* 4 to 8 pm aggravation) point directly to the remedy. The concomitants are also of significant value. *Mental concomitants are important in physical diseases and physical concomitants are important in mental diseases.* The mental concomitants like irritability, weeping and fear etc. are good indicators of specific acute remedies.

In acute cases with symptom deficiency, any of the above mentioned elements might be the sole criteria for prescribing. At times difficulty arising out of lack of characteristics can be overcome by concentrating on the location, e.g. *Colocynthis* in abdominal pain, *Merc.* group in throat affections and tonsillitis and *Thlaspi bursa pestoris* in uterine haemorrhages. Such remedies are called as organ remedies. According to James Compton Burnett, the well-known organ remedies are employed on indications provided by the location and type of pathological changes.

A recent cause responsible for appearance of acute complaints often helps in acute prescribing. For example, *Ignatia amara* in complaints after death in the family, *Cantharis vesicatoria* in complaints after burns in household accidents, occipital headache with vertigo after a fearful experience or fright indicates *Gelsemium sempervirens* etc. The physical causative factors may be useful at times, e.g. backache after a prolonged journey indicates *Bellis perennis*.

Dr. K.N. Kasad has advanced the concept of 'Fixed General Totality' that needs to be taken into account along with complaints at the level of particulars or sectors. According to him, first there is a generalized disturbance in the evolution of acute diseases. It manifests as the general totality. This general totality remains the same and does not change hence it is called 'Fixed General Totality.' Thus, the acute totality consists of fixed general totality plus the totality of the sector involved. Usually the precipitating cause, general modalities, physical generals and changes in mental state are taken under this fixed totality. The sector totality changes with the part or sector affected. Sector totality consists of location, sensation, modalities and concomitants.

In acute diseases the chronic or constitutional symptoms of the patient seem to disappear. The vital force brings forth the acute symptomatology, therefore acute symptoms are prominently seen. The acute symptoms disappear when treated with a suitable acute remedy and the previously submerged chronic symptoms reappear. It is the time when the indicated constitutional remedy should be prescribed to prevent relapses.

According to Dr. Kasad, constitutional remedy sometimes needs to be given in acute diseases. This is done when the vital force is not able to throw up acute symptoms and the generals become prominent instead of going into background. If the constitutional remedy is not given at this point the case may turn fatal. Constitutional remedy can abort the acute disease if prescribed in the prodromal phase. In case of an epidemic, the remedy is selected on the basis of characteristic symptoms collected from first few cases. This remedy proves curative only in that particular epidemic. A new *'genius epidemicus'* needs to be selected if a similar epidemic happens next year. This is because each epidemic has its own unique totality that varies from the previous one. The epidemic specific proves 'prophylactic' if given to other members of patient's family.

The knowledge of the constitutional remedy of the patient is sometimes one of the quickest aids in acute prescribing in homeopathic practice. Thus, the throat complaints of a *Calc. carb* patient will call for *Belladonna* more often, while the acute complaints of *Silicea* lady would often require *Pulsatilla*.

II. CHRONIC PRESCRIBING

The particulars are more important in acute prescribing and the generals indicating the constitution of the patient are vital in chronic prescribing. Proper perception of evolutionary totality is essential in chronic prescribing. The selected remedy must resemble with patient's mental makeup, miasmatic background, physical generals and diathesis, etc. One should not get worried about wrong selection if the remedy does not cover little particulars. The generals are all important.

At times in a chronic case with advanced pathology there is lack of clear-cut indications for the chronic constitutional remedy. Such cases have paucity of characteristics. The striking pathological condition indicates the remedy in such cases. It needs to be prescribed frequently in low potencies.

Most of the times in infants and children especially neonates, there are no indications for constitutional remedy because the constitutional features require time to evolve during growth of the child. In such cases knowledge of constitutional remedy of the parents is very often helpful in determining the chronic remedy. The constitutional remedy especially of the mother forms a reliable basis for chronic prescribing.

Remedy relationships may prove helpful in chronic prescription. A physician can proceed from acute remedy to the chronic one after a careful study of the remedy relationships. Boenninghausen's Therapeutic Pocket Book can provide the most reliable help in this regard.

Sometimes nosodes may be indicated in chronic prescribing on the basis of symptom similarity. The chronic cases with mixed up symptomatology make the prescribing difficult on account of changes and alternating of symptom groups. Such cases should be analysed from the miasmatic standpoint and nosodes can be used to clear up the case and restore the sensitivity of the patient to constitutional remedy.

Intercurrent remedies are prescribed in a chronic case when the action of a well-selected constitutional remedy gets blocked and the patient refuses to make further progress. In such cases analysis of the case from miasmatic point of view indicates the type of miasm responsible for this block and accordingly a suitable anti-miasmatic remedy is prescribed to remove it.

INFERENCE

Although, remedy selection depends on many factors like physician's knowledge of materia medica, allied sciences, his ability to perceive totality, and the amount and type of information available in a case, still unprejudiced thinking is must as faulty thinking leads to faulty prescription. At times, for a novice and even for a physician with sufficient experience, it is difficult to keep the thinking in right direction. There is always a chance of committing mistakes in prescribing, hence self-assessment from time to time is necessary. It is hard to find a homeopath who has never committed a mistake in remedy selection. Some techniques of prescribing can be used in remedy selection without departing from principles. A homeopath should not forget that totality is the only formula of prescribing in homeopathy. There is no short cut for gaining mastery over remedy selection.

However, from the above discussion we can conclude that although remedy selection is an art that has to be consciously developed by every physician, still some basic guidelines based on homeopathic philosophy can be formulated to guide our thinking in right direction. Thinking along scientific lines (i.e. with principles and laws of homeopathic philosophy) can only prevent us from making bizarre prescriptions, keeping our thought process on track and thus decreasing the possibility of errors or rather 'blunders' in prescribing.

■

CHAPTER 12

Miasmatic Diagnosis

- ❖ Evolution of Miasmatic Theory   258
- ❖ Scientific Foundations of Miasmatic Theory   261
- ❖ Miasmatic Diagnosis   262
- ❖ Comparative Table of Miasms   266

CHAPTER 12

MIASMATIC DIAGNOSIS

Every homeopath at one time or the other has observed that some patients return with the same symptomatology after a brief interval of disappearance of symptoms. This happens inspite of prescribing the most similar remedy. In such a situation majority of homeopaths repeat the same remedy or prescribe the same with some alteration. The result is still the same, temporary relief followed by a relapse. This is precisely the situation which led Hahnemann to the discovery of miasms. Today homeopaths seem to have conveniently forgotten this fact. A large majority neglects the miasmatic background of the case. They never care to diagnose the miasm in the case and hence the remedy selected does not meet the predominant miasm in the case. This leads to reappearance of symptoms after a temporary disappearance. Practitioners who reject the miasmatic theory as being non-essential part of homeopathic practice often meet with this situation in their private practice. The other section of homeopathic physicians, those who believe in miasmatic theory have a problem too. They fail to apply the theory in practice. Homeopathic literature since Hahnemann's time talks volumes about miasms but seldom do we find clear-cut guidelines regarding application of miasmatic theory.

Amongst the believers in miasmatic theory there is a disagreement with regard to interpretation, explanation and application of miasmatic theory. Their condition is not any different from the one described in the well-known story of five blindfolded men trying to describe an elephant. The current discussion aims to understand the evolution and scientific basis of miasmatic theory. An attempt to determine the utility of miasmatic theory in management of chronic case is also done. It is hoped that this discussion would sufficiently clarify the matter and help the reader in utilizing it in clinical practice.

EVOLUTION OF MIASMATIC THEORY

Hahnemann's inability to fit the results of application of single remedy within the definition of cure, which he advanced, led him to discovery of the theory of chronic miasms. Hahnemann had already defined cure as permanent disappearance of symptoms. He was disappointed to find only a temporary removal of symptoms (recovery) in his practice. Whatever he did with the remedies in his early days of practice by application of law of similars only relieved but did not cure. Hahnemann having a very keen, logical and inquiring mind was not ready to accept this. He had to prove that either the law of similars is totally wrong, partially wrong or may be that it is curative only in certain diseases and not in others. The other possibility could be that the definition of cure itself is incorrect. He was not prepared to bargain for either.

For over a period of 11 years Hahnemann studied his patients and their complaints. He collected the data, searched the facts and classified the facts or symptoms. He classified the diseases as:

1. Acute Diseases.
2. Chronic Diseases.

He excluded from his classification episodes of accidents, injuries, poisonings and those conditions readily explainable on the basis of mechanical factors, since in all these conditions the vital dynamis had little role to play and these conditions did not call for true medicinal intervention according to law of similars.

Hahnemann concluded that acute diseases were brought on by unfavourable factors in the external environment, which were easily identifiable and hence removable. Their removal brought on cure. Application of homeopathic remedies selected on the basis of similarity helped greatly in the process of recovery and cure in these diseases. The acute diseases had a short course and would either end in death or cure.

The other type i.e. chronic diseases had features suggesting that they could not be termed acute. After a careful study of symptomatology and past history Hahnemann grouped these cases in to two categories,

(a) Patients with no history of venereal infection
(b) Patients with history of venereal infection of syphilis and gonorrhoea.

The first category of patients gave a history of itching skin manifestation suppressed by local treatment. The complaints of these patients started since that period. According to Hahnemann these suppressions produced the miasm 'Psora.' This Psora affected the vital force adversely and led to predisposition to diseases and complaints in these patients. He called these patients 'Psoric.' In the second category the venereal diseases were suppressed by local measures. These suppressions produced the miasms 'Syphillis' and 'Sycosis' respectively. He labeled these patients as 'Syphilitic' and 'Sycotic.' The remedies useful for correcting these states were called Anti-syphillitic and Anti-sycotic remedies. Hahnemann investigated the problem posed to him in depth keeping in mind the wider view. Therefore, in his investigation he paid special attention to all that happened in the personal as well as the family history of the patient. His views evolved steadily from 1790 to 1810. He realized that his prescription was based on precipitating cause. It was natural because in those times cause was not classified. Cause was thought of as merely something that precedes the onset of disease symptoms. Hahnemann's classification of patient's symptomatology revealed to him that cause could be recent or remote. The remote cause or the root of disease is what is interfering with the process of cure. Thus, he concluded that miasms were the cause of chronic diseases. The existence of miasms hinders the process of cure. So, the miasms can be regarded as the gulf between recovery and cure.

The term miasm was used by Hahnemann to describe the defect in the constitution that caused the reappearance of symptoms. After Hahnemann propounded the theory of miasms, he regarded the acute diseases as expressions of latent Psora and recommended that patients with acute diseases should be managed by acute remedies and subsequently, in the quiescent phase, be given Antipsorics to build up their resistance so that relapses do not occur. All these observations of Hahnemann were published in *The Chronic Diseases.*

Hahnemann grouped various symptoms and pathological conditions into three broad groups. We can conclude that Hahnemann's theory of chronic miasms was an attempt at generalization and classification of both the patients and the drugs into three groups, i.e. Psoric, Syphilitic, and Sycotic. Therefore, we can say that Hahnemann's miasms and general pathology are two sides of the same coin. We should avoid confusing the miasms with the clinical states from which they were supposed to have arisen. The term 'miasm' is employed to denote the cause as well as the effect. For example, Psora, Syphilis and Sycosis are used to denote the causative miasms as well as their effects, the respective grouping of syndromes.

After Hahnemann, many stalwarts added their own observations and opinions to the miasmatic theory. Each one applied different logic to explain the miasms. Allen added the fourth group i.e. Tubercular, which according to him was a combination of Psora and Syphilis. Stuart Close studied miasms from the bacteriological angle and co-related bacteriology with miasms. Roberts advanced the theory that miasms are deficiency of essential elements. Dr. Dhawale had tried to co-relate all these theories. He defines miasm as the susceptibility of the wrong order. According to him four miasms are four types of susceptibilities or constitutions having predisposition to type of diseases and conditions classified under each miasm. He studied the miasms by adding the time dimension and described the evolution from Psora to Syphilis with the intervening phases of Sycosis and Tubercular miasm.

Today our knowledge of pathology is far more advanced due to discovery of various modern investigative procedures and machinery. Any pathological condition can be detected right when the changes have just begun. Therefore, we should try to interpret each miasm in the light of our current knowledge of pathology. Classification of various diseases and conditions under various miasms done in Hahnemann's time would not be the same today considering our present day knowledge of pathology. A variation in classification is permitted as long as it can be logically co-related with the basics of each miasm.

SCIENTIFIC FOUNDATIONS OF MIASMATIC THEORY

Science is a general term used to describe and categorize different theories, phenomenon and principles. There are various types or levels of science. A science can be applied, fundamental, descriptive, etc. Homeopathy is a science based on experiment. It is experimental clinical medicine. Therefore, homeopathy and its various theories have to be judged on these grounds. Any other way of evaluating homeopathic theories is illogical. The theory of miasms was deduced logically and established experimentally. This is the first reason why the miasmatic theory can be regarded as scientific. To establish the scientific basis of miasmatic theory, the criteria that need to be fulfilled to call a theory or principle scientific must be defined. The criteria that are required to be fulfilled (as stated by Dr. J.N. Kanjilal) to establish the scientific basis of a theory are as follows:

1. The theory or principle must be based on clearly observed data, facts and phenomena.
2. It must be repeatedly confirmed by future observations and experiences under similar conditions.
3. It must give clear and correct guidance in anticipating the future events.

All these criteria are fulfilled by the theory of miasms; hence, it can be regarded as having a scientific basis.

MIASMATIC DIAGNOSIS

DEFINITION

The miasms are the types of predispositions to illness or morbid susceptibilities or the defects in the constitution brought about through hereditary genetic influence. The presence of each miasm can be identified by virtue of the attributes or characteristics of each miasm in the patient. In all the patients a homeopath would find a part of all three pathological characteristics. In spite of that, at any given point of time only one of them will always be dominant determining and modulating the type of disease expressions in the patient. Miasms are the various stages in the evolution of an individual from being a healthy person to a patient as he is today.

The disappearance of characteristics of one stage is followed by the appearance of the next.

Thus, miasmatic diagnosis can be defined as identifying or perceiving the miasm (or miasms) expressing itself through various symptoms and disease conditions at the moment the patient comes under a homeopath's observation.

This diagnosis would indicate to a physician the activity of a certain miasm or he might discover a total mix-up in the picture due to blending of various miasms, hence classification cannot be done.

According to Dr. M.L. Dhawale miasmatic diagnosis involves two stages:

1. Identification of the fundamental miasm, which is indicated by the family history of diseases as well as the personal, past history.
2. Identifying the dominant miasm deduced from a consideration of the prominent expressions of disease (or characteristics in the case) at the time of observation.

It is necessary to comprehend the significance of every part of what is meant by 'Miasmatic Diagnosis' to ensure that it is implemented in the right spirit. A clear understanding of this concept would also insure that the confusion over miasms and miasmatic diagnosis that we have so far been used to is dispelled.

Dr. Dhawale states that, "Each constitution is an admixture of all the four miasms as is evident from the full blown disease expressions revealed in the homeopathic materia medica. At the same time we discover in this unfolding a tendency to favour expressions in a differential manner, favouring one miasm over the rest. Similar favouring is also seen in the phase of diathesis.

He attempts to clarify the process of miasmatic diagnosis by stating that, "We need to be clear that the four miasms are never seen in actual practice, since they are abstractions. What we actually see in patients is a mixture of the various symptoms according to a distinctive individual plan that has unfolded over a period of time. This is an expression of the past (familial as well as personal) interacting with the various environmental factors from time to time to give rise to the evolutionary picture of the disease. This picture, on analysis permits us to derive the expressions of the four miasms on the strength of certain criteria we have laid down for each."

To summarise the issue we can conclude that a patient's case record is an evolutionary display of the illness. It indicates the way in which various miasms got activated from time to time in response to environmental factors, giving rise to a fine blending of miasmatic expressions. None of the miasms get terminated at any single point of time. The expressions of miasmatic forces in a patient's case record are variable. Accurate miasmatic diagnosis, therefore, requires skills of analysis and differentiation to bring out the specific contribution of each miasm in giving rise to individual picture of disease.

NEED FOR MIASMATIC DIAGNOSIS

The followers of Hahnemann like Hughes and Dr. Hering rejected the miasmatic theory. They were of the opinion that as long as a homeopath selects his remedy on the basis of symptom similarity there is no need of adopting or rejecting the miasmatic theory. Hering believed that miasmatic theory is of no value and has no influence in treating patients. Symptom similarity is the only requirement of treating patients with homeopathy.

Allen logically defended the theory stating that one cannot select a true Simillimum unless one is able to perceive or identify the predominant miasm in the case. Only a true Simillimum can cure the patient. Therefore, a remedy that is not similar to the miasmatic background of the case would not cure. This makes it necessary for a homeopath to perceive the miasmatic background of each patient in order to select the miasmatic Simillimum.

An allopath cannot treat a fever without diagnosing it as malaria or typhoid. An ayurvedic practitioner would not treat a case without identifying the predominance of 'Vata' 'Pitta' and 'Kapha' (the three 'doshas') and the patients 'Prakruti' or constitution. Similarly a homeopath cannot treat a patient curatively without perceiving the predominant miasm in the case. He must find out whether his patient is psoric, sycotic, syphilitic or tubercular or has blending of two or three miasms in order to select the true simillimum. When a physician prescribes a constitutional remedy keeping in view the predominant miasmatic expressions in the case, such a constitutional remedy removes the presenting symptoms and the process of cure extends further to the removal of the entire abnormal susceptibility so that all tendency to recurrence is eliminated. Identification of dominant miasm in the case serves as a compass to guide the homeopath in his journey from recovery to cure.

Advantages of Miasmatic Diagnosis

1. It helps the homeopath in detection of constitutional tendencies (even in pre-clinical stage of the disease).
2. He has the advantage of making a clinical diagnosis even in prodromal stage.
3. It greatly helps in curative as well as preventive management of cases.

The advantages of miasmatic diagnosis according to *Dr. Proceso Sanchez Ortega* are as follows:

1. It spares us the failure of supposing that we are going to cure when we are scarcely going to succeed in a relative and fleeting alleviation of the symptoms.

2. It enables us to understand the profound pathology which we must inevitably confront sooner or later and which is our duty to bring to the surface, so that it will be accessible to the correct treatment seeking a true cure.

3. It gives us an unshakeable basis for a relative prognosis of the case, considered in all its profundity and going into the constitutional miasmatic factors which have determined the series of dysfunctions and lesions: the patient's behaviour, traits as presented in his biopathography, that is, not only in his pathological history but also in the different aspects of his life — physical development, sickness, attitudes and conduct at various stages of his life (childhood, puberty, adolescence, etc.). Also his achievements, frustrations, tendencies, pleasures, vices, loves and preferences in social life.

COMPARATIVE TABLE OF MIASMS

The following table would help in easy understanding and comparison of the four miasmatic types. Every case has numerous expressions belonging to various miasms, therefore the patient's data also needs to be transferred to similar type of table putting each expression in the case, to the miasm it belongs. Tabulation of patient's data helps in finding out the dominant miasm in the case so that treatment can be directed accordingly.

The following table incorporates the individualizing features of each miasmatic type at various levels. It is based on Dr. J. H. Allen and Dr. M. L. Dhawale's work on miasms.

TABLE OF MIASMS

(Based on Dr. J. H. Allen and Dr. M. L. Dhawale's work on miasms)

Feature	PSORA	SYCOSIS	TUBERCULAR	SYPHILIS
Type of Activity	Hyperactivity (Vasomotor and sympathetic), uncontrolled	Slow, inactivity, inertia	**HYPERACTIVITY**, erratic type, changeable	Violent, uncontrolled
Type of Response	Hypersensitive, quick, alert, active, acute, sudden intense, exaggerated	Slow, sluggish, inefficient, inappropriate, remote (aberrant immune responses), wandering, slow recovery.	Quick, hyperdynamic alternating, erratic, changeable	Violent, destructive, disproportionate, irrational
Metabolism	Rapid, assimilation poor, mal-absorption, malnutrition.	Slow, tardy, inefficient metabolic adjustments (Cetabolism diminished, Anabolism +++), retention.	Rapid, assimilation poor, anabolism decreased, Cetabolism+++.	Rapid, assimilation, poor, anabolism decreased.

Feature	PSORA	SYCOSIS	TUBERCULAR	SYPHILIS
Diathesis		Gouty-rheumatic, uric acid diathesis	Haemorrhagic	Irreversible, structural
Type of Pathology	Functional (minimal structural alteration), reversible, simple inflammation without suppuration, swelling	Hypertrophy, tumours (benign), retention, excessive growths, edema	Easy abscess (delayed healing), sinus formation, fibrosis, scarring, calcification, hemorrhage, lymphadenopathy	Alterations, degeneration, decay, deformities, ulceration, caries
Type of Pathology	Congestion vesicular eruptions	RES Aberrations Deposition (Accumulation) metastasis, remote inflammatory non-suppurative cysts, warts	**Infections** (due to reduced resistance), fissures, cracks, suppuration	Necrosis, atrophy, malignant tumors, premature senile, changes, cracks, fissures, fibrosis

Feature	PSORA	SYCOSIS	TUBERCULAR	SYPHILIS
Diseases	Labile hypertension, nocturnal enuresis, dyspepsia, chicken pox, scabies, low blood pressure, low blood glucose, thyrotoxicosis without goiter, impotence, sterility, functional uterine disorders, difficult dentition, vaginismus, malnutrition, malabsorption, nervous break-down	Obesity, auto-immune disorders, allergic disorders, asthma, chronic simple bronchitis, SLE, gout, rheumatism, anemia, colics, moles, sebaceous cysts, renal calculi, thyrotoxicosis with goitre, toxemia of pregnancy, abnormal growth of hair	Diabetes, bleeding gums, hemorrhagic disorders, hernia, piles, bacterial and viral infections (protracted recovery from infections), parasitic infestations (worms, amebiasis) tonsillitis, measles, Crohn's disease, Hodgkin's disease, Beryllium poisoning, dental caries, tooth decay, premature greying of hair	Alopecia, cataract, osteoarthritis ankylosis, gangrene, atherosclerosis, IHD, marasmus, easy sprains, retinosis, pigmentosa, coppery eruptions, malignancies, leucoderma
Organs & Tissues Affected (Site) Factors	SKIN (envelops), (upper layers), mucous membranes,	SKIN (deeper layers, sebaceous glands),	BONES, RESPIRATORY ORGANS,	Cartilage, Bones, Teeth

Feature	PSORA	SYCOSIS	TUBERCULAR	SYPHILIS
	MIND, UTERUS, NERVOUS SYSTEM, ENDOCRINE GLANDS, suppression of skin eruptions, normal discharges (like perspiration), emotions, excitement, grief, sorrow, fear	SOFT ORGANS & Tissues (Prominently affected), Joints, Muscles, KIDNEYS, LIVER, GOUT, suppression of abnormal discharges	Blood Vessels, Glands, GIT, Sexual Organs, poor resistance, hectic activity, poor resources, poor reaction	Mucus membranes, eyes, suppression of abnormal discharges
Modalities	< Before menses < Morning < New moon < Motion < Exertion < Odours < Touch > Rest, lying down > Heat (pains) > Free eliminations	< Damp, getting wet < Daytime < Meat < Natural eliminations (Sweat, urine, stool) < Rest < Change of weather > Slow motion > lying on abdomen > Dry weather	< Cold < Change of weather to cold < Exertion < Evening < Bathing < Working in water < Washing (skin) < Sunday (headache) > Haemorrhages	< Rest < Storms < Night < Artificial light < Cold & heat < Natural eliminations (stool urine sweat) > Motion > Cold applications

Feature	PSORA	SYCOSIS	TUBERCULAR	SYPHILIS
	(perspiration, urination, diarrhoea) > Return of suppressed skin manifestations	> Return of Suppressed normal discharges (menses) > Bending double > Hard pressure (colics)		
Mental Make-up (Mind)	Keen intellect, quick perception, memory+++ mental faculties alert, active, hypersensitive, emotional, anxious, fearful, restless, poor concentration, competent but fears failure	Dull intellect, poor memory, perception poor, confusion, fixed ideas, anticipatory, anxiety, agitational anxiety, fear of failure (without awareness of competence), guilt, insecurity, fear of death, suspicious, jealous, envious, hatred, delusions, illusions and hallucinations,	Keen intellect, memory +++, heightened perception, E.S.P., clairvoyance, weak will, motivation poor, insecurity, fright strong, desires and attachments, fancies & fantasies, swings of mood, changeable temperament, behaviour nervous, irritability and excitability	Slow comprehension, perception poor decision making poor, moral depravity, stubborn, morose, guilt-complexes, fixed ideas, hatred, violent uncontrolled anger, violence in action, psychopathic personality,

Feature	PSORA	SYCOSIS	TUBERCULAR	SYPHILIS
		brooding, hypochondriac, violence in thought		manic, psychosis, cruel, cunning, mean minded, vindictive
Sensations and Complaints	Dryness, "Sensations as if", ravenous hunger (all gone sensation), alternating states, hot flushes, ebullitions, deficiency disorders, skin: dry, itching, rough, dirty, unwashed looking, < open air, < evening, > scratching, burning, headache < sun, cold > heat, rest, craving sweets, diarrohoea >	Stiffness, soreness, lameness, spasms, colics, greenish sour acrid discharges, mottling of mucous membranes, anemia, skin: oily, greasy, spots, warty growths, pains < cold damp weather, < lying down > pressure > bending double.	Ravenous hunger with emaciation, haemorrhage, abscess and sinus formation, cheesy, bloody, musty, mouldy discharges, skin: cracked, fissured, pustular, scars breakdown, fair complexion & silken eyelashes, premature greying of hair, white spots on nails, generalized lymphadenopathy, recurrent infections, craving tobacco, tea	Band sensation, offensive perspiration, weak joints — easy sprains, glandular affections, skin: copper coloured or brownish eruptions, thick heavy scales, eruptions esp. about joints, flexures of body in circular rings, bores the head into pillow and rolls from side to side

CHAPTER 13

Fundamentals of Potency Selection

- ❖ Evolution of Theory of 'Small Dose' and 'Potency'   275
- ❖ Susceptibility and 'Susceptibility-Potency' Interrelationship   279
- ❖ Laws of Potency Selection   284
- ❖ Potency Types in Centesimal Scale   285
- ❖ Scientific Basis of Potency Selection   285

CHAPTER 13

FUNDAMENTALS OF POTENCY SELECTION

Choice of remedy based on similarity insures amelioration of symptoms but only similarity at symptomatic level is not enough, as the speed of recovery largely depends on the potency selected. True similarity is, therefore, the similarity of the drug to patients image along with the similarity of the dose and repetition. We should rather aim at selecting the 'potential simillimum' which assumes much significance owing to its bearing on the pace of amelioration of symptoms. A potential simillimum guarantees faster amelioration of symptoms without unwanted aggravation. The aggravation induced by it is so small that it is hardly perceptible and hence a true homeopathic aggravation. Considering its important role in recovery of the patient, it becomes mandatory that we select the potency accurately.

EVOLUTION OF THEORY OF 'SMALL DOSE' AND 'POTENCY'

Before one proceed to the fundamentals of potency selection it is essential to know the path of exploration followed by

Hahnemann especially with reference to the development of the concept of dose and dynamization in the formative years of homeopathy. In the year 1790 the foundation stone of homeopathy was laid by proving of Peruvian bark and from 1790 to 1796 Hahnemann was involved in applying the principle of similia, without any special attention to the size of doses.

In his pre-homeopathic medical career his dosing of medicines was similar to his colleagues. In his article *'Directions for Cure of Old Sores and Ulcers'* in the year 1784 (four years before the proving of Peruvian bark) he writes of (prescribing with allopathic standards) antimony in doses of 5-50 grams and Jalap root in 20-70 grains. This is a historical evidence of the fact that in 1790 he prescribed Cinchona according to allopathic standards of that time, at 1 to 2 ounces (45-75 grams) per 24 hours. During his experiments of treating with the similia principle, he came to know that a well-chosen simillimum could act in a rather small dose. In the year 1796 in his *'Essay on a New Principle for Ascertaining the Curative Powers of Drugs'* for the first time he makes reference to the use of "small doses" but does not clarify this any further.

By the year 1798 Hahnemann started using small crude doses homeopathically. Although these small doses were still rather large as compared to later homeopathic standards, but we can surely say that they represent dramatic reductions from the allopathic size of doses which his colleagues used at that time. Serial dilutions appeared on the homeopathic scene for the first time in the year 1799. In this year in his booklet *'Cure and Prevention of Scarlet Fever'* which was actually published in 1801 Hahnemann gives detailed statements regarding dilution. At this point, we don't find any trace of trituration and succussion. In this booklet, Hahnemann gives descriptions of mixing such as *"shaking the whole well"* and *"intimately mixed...by shaking it for a minute."* It shows his interest in dispersing the drug substance well throughout the medium of dilution. His understanding of dilutions, attenuations or reduced doses at that time can be seen in the terms he uses to describe these preparations such as *"weak solution of belladonna."*

Reference to Hahnemann's case notes at this point suggest that he was moving to "infinitesimal" doses and had began to appreciate the ability of the extreme dilutions. But for his assertions on the efficacy of such "infinitesimal" doses he received criticism from his contemporaries, to which he responded through his article in Hufeland's Journal in 1801. By this time he appreciated the release of medicinal powers by dispersal of a substance in a quantity of solute. But in his 1801 article *"On the Power of Small Doses of Medicines in General and of Belladonna in Particular"* there was no actual mention of the notion of potentization or dynamization of remedies. In the 2 volume *'Fragmenta de Veribus Medicamentorum Positivis'* published in 1805 as well as in part I of Materia Medica Pura which came in 1811 there is no mention of dose.

But in first edition of Organon published in 1810 he referred only to "small doses" individually determined for each medicine. In the second edition in 1819 the paragraphs 300 to 308 were devoted to the issue of dose. Here he states, "The suitability of a medicine for any given case of illness depends not only on a relevant homeopathic selection, but just as much the correct quantity necessary or rather the smallness of the dose." He went on to suggest that dose determination requires "clear experiments, careful observation and accurate experience." In 1812 epidemic of intermittent fever, he employed *Arnica* in 18th centesimal dilution and *Nux vomica* in the 9th centesimal dilution or potency.

Historical references suggest that it is in the year 1825 Hahnemann actually began viewing his preparations as "dynamizations" (dynamische) or "potentizations"(potenz, potenzirung) rather than mere dilutions or attenuations. In his article "Information for the Truth Seeker" published in the same year he writes that by trituration the latent medicinal power is wonderfully liberated and vitalized, as if once freed from the fetters of matter, it could act upon the human organism more insistently and fully. In the year 1835 in part two of 1st edition of 'Chronic Diseases' he gave a detailed description of the process of trituration, mainly for the first 3 centesimal dilutions of insoluble medicinal substances. At this point of time, some of his followers like General Korsakoff in Russia & Dr. Schreter in Lemberg went on to develop higher and higher potencies and General Korsakoff went up to 1500th centesimal potency. In response to which Hahnemann wrote to Korsakoff & Schreter urging them to adopt 30 c as the limit or as a standard potency.

In 3rd edition of Organon published in 1833 Hahnemann clearly spells out the concept of potentization/dynamization in aphorism 269 and aphorisms 270-271. In this edition, he only falls slightly short of recommending 30 c potency as a standard. About the same time i.e. 1832 he started experimenting with olfaction of remedies which he has described in his preface to Boenninghausen's 'List of Symptoms of the Antipsoric Medicines' (Repertory of Antipsoric Medicines) and in 5th edition of Organon. Year 1838 (just five years before his death) saw Hahnemann developing the LM (fifty millesimal) potency scale which was referred to as his *"medicaments au globule."* At the time of his death his remedy chest contained 888 vials of centesimal remedies in 6th, 18th, 24th & 30th centesimal potencies & a few bottles of 200th centesimal potency, and 1716 vials of LM potencies, with few major polycrests stoked up to LM 30. Hahnemann used all degrees of dilution, low as well as high, as the individual case required. Taking into consideration his approach to potency based on the demands of the case, every true homeopath should also select the potency according to the demands of the case. He should be open to all potency types.

Fundamentals of Potency Selection

How to select potency is the next important question about which we do not find much guidance in Hahnemann's writings. Unfortunately it still remains the most perplexing part of homeopathic practice that has to be dealt with everyday by a physician. The reason for this seems to be the vague guidelines in philosophical texts which leave much to be desired. Many neophytes are in total dark when it comes to choice of potency and gaining mastery over it is a matter of experience. While for others it is conceptually quite clear but too difficult in application. But a physician who knows the fundamentals of potency selection has less trouble in selecting the right potency than the one who depends on 'experiences' in daily practice.

One of the very basic concepts which is closely linked with the issue of potency selection is the concept of 'Susceptibility.' We find only three aphorisms i.e. 30, 31, 32 in Organon of Medicine where Hahnemann makes a passing reference to the susceptibility. As the selection of potency for every case largely depends on the susceptibility of the patient it is very essential to understand the concept of susceptibility first, followed by a clear perception of the 'susceptibility – potency' interrelationship.

SUSCEPTIBILITY AND 'SUSCEPTIBILITY-POTENCY' INTERRELATIONSHIP

The meaning of the term 'Environment' assumes great importance in understanding the concept of susceptibility. Environment can be defined as the aggregate of external and internal conditions that have influence on the life and development of organism or individual (human being). Environment can be of two types:

1. Internal Environment.
2. External Environment.

1. INTERNAL ENVIRONMENT

It pertains to each and every component part of every tissue and organ and their harmonious functioning in the body. There is a continual adjustment and readjustment in the human mechanism to keep itself in physiological balance or dynamic equilibrium. This steady state of human environment of the body is called "Homeostasis" by the physiologists.

2. EXTERNAL ENVIRONMENT

It includes all external circumstances and conditions of the individual which have got effect on the development and life of an individual. If the external environment is favourable to an individual he can make full use of physical and mental capacities he has inherited provided internal environment is in order. The external environment of an individual comprises of three closely related components:

(a) Physical Environment.
(b) Biological Environment.
(c) Social Environment.

Every individual right from its birth starts interacting with environment. The environment is affecting the individual by sending or producing various stimuli at all times. In order to maintain a normal equilibrium or balance the individual has to respond in such a manner that he adjusts himself and adopts himself to environment.

That is necessary for maintaining normalcy without getting adversely affected by various disturbing stimuli. The inherent capacity in an individual to receive and react to the stimuli in the environment is known as susceptibility. It is the fundamental quality of all the living things. It is made known to the observer through the responses or the reactions that occur when the host meets the

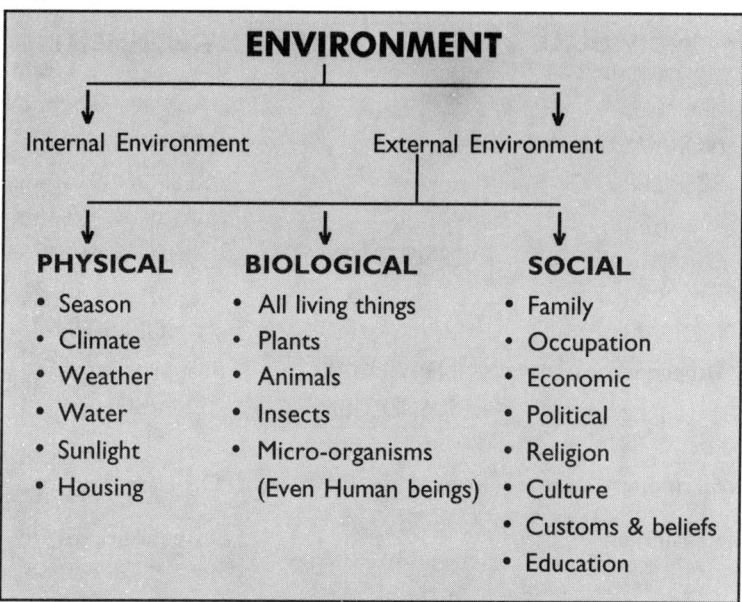

environment. In other words the individual-environment interactions in totality constitute susceptibility. As already stated it is expressed through responses which in turn depend on the sensitivity. If the sensitivity is normal the responses are normal or appropriate and the equilibrium of the system is not disturbed. It means that susceptibility is normal. If the sensitivity is abnormal the responses too are abnormal and the abnormal responses in turn lead to disturbed balance of the system and lead to what we call disease. The responses are abnormal, inappropriate and inadequate to meet the challenges posed by the disturbing stimuli when either the stimuli are stronger or the sensitivity is increased or decreased (i.e. abnormal sensitivity).

The type of sensitivity of every individual is determined by one very important factor, the genetic pattern or the hereditary plan. The hereditary background and the genetic pattern vary from individual to individual and hence the type of sensitivity to various stimuli also varies. Thus the response to same stimuli is different

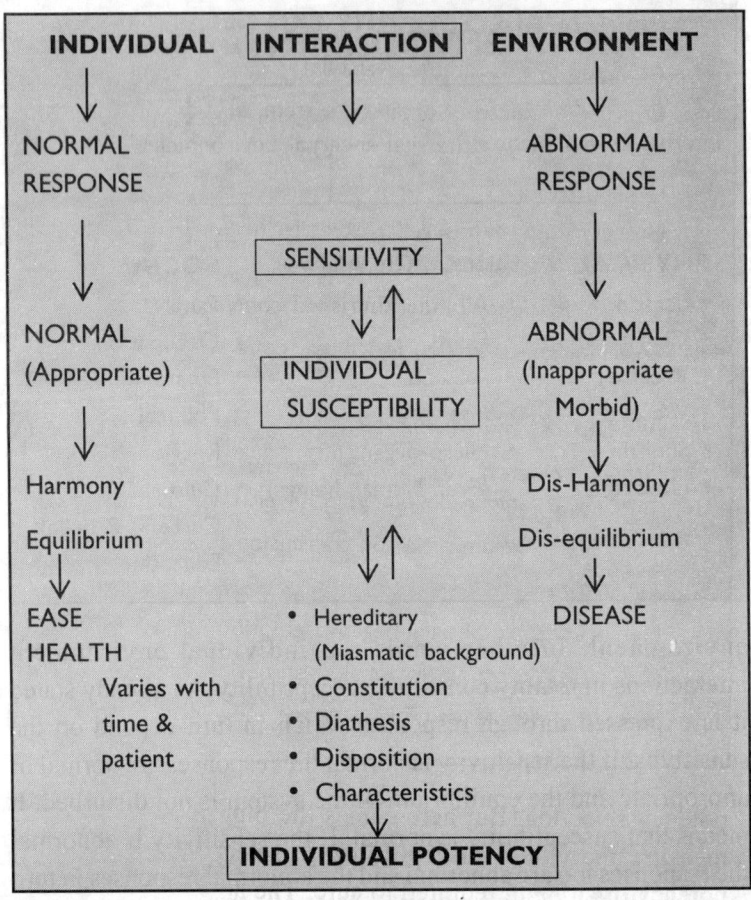

in different individuals or in other words the susceptibility to a particular stimulus differs or varies from individual to individual. So we can conclude that, the potency required to meet this 'individual susceptibility' also differs with every individual and hence every case needs a different potency.

Thus, the concept of susceptibility (especially individual susceptibility) and potency selection (potency required to meet the individual susceptibility) are inseparable & interdependent, infact measurement of individual susceptibility is the backbone of

> **ABNORMAL SUSCEPTIBILITY CAN DEVELOP FROM:**
> (As stated by Dr. Sarabhai Kapadia)
> - Overuse or abuse of organ or system. (These things exhaust, pervert or thwart the vital energy.)
> - Mechanical injury.
> - Unaccustomed exposure (to excessive heat or cold or exposure to sudden variations of temperature).
> - Dietary deficiency (undernourished condition).
> - Overindulgence in rich food, tea, coffee, alcohol and other stimulants.
> - Antimalarials and wormicides.
> - Drugs (containing sulphur, coal tar derivatives, heavy metals, mercury, arsenic, cadmium, gold, silver, tin etc.).
> - Vaccination, Serum or Blood transfusion.
> - Air pollution.
> - Mental stress (especially negative emotions).
> - Sexual dissatisfaction (for prolonged periods).
> - Miasmatic complexes (Psora, sycosis and syphilis).

potency selection. But here comes the bigger problem. How to measure individual susceptibility to select the corresponding potency or strength required to cure. The answer is not difficult. We know that individual susceptibility is nothing but the totality of individual sensitivity and hence the sensitivity expressed at various levels is the scale to measure the susceptibility. One must not forget that potency of a remedy is actually the measure or form of energy stored in the remedy or it is the strength or the degree of ability to act on the same plane or in the same depth at which disease is expressed or expressing itself. So a remedy (going by the modus operandi of homeopathic cures) would produce the artificial disease of same kind or same degree or same strength only if the degree of individual susceptibility matches with the degree of potency employed. If the potency is lower or higher than required, it is not in the same plane and hence lacks the ability to affect the individual at the same depth as the disease and hence inadequate or insufficient. This would mean that if the potency is not right the remedy is only similar at the symptomatic level but would not be a complete simillimum or potential simillimum and hence rapid, gentle and permanent cure cannot be expected. Therefore the potency must be right. Appropriate potency when employed leads to quick recovery because the amount of drug energy meets the individual demands. An individual exhibits maximum susceptibility to the simillimum. Actually the administration of simillimum leads to better adaptation by satisfying the increased susceptibility (seen in disease) and lowering it to fall within the limits of normality.

LAWS OF POTENCY SELECTION

On the basis of the logical interpretation and the logical correlation between the concept of susceptibility and potency that has been attempted above some laws of potency selection can be formulated which are as follows:

1. Susceptibility being constant variable the potency required for each case cannot be constant.
2. Degree of sensitivity is directly proportional to the level of susceptibility and the level of susceptibility in turn is directly proportional to the degree of potency required.
3. Susceptibility is inversely proportional to the degree of pathological changes, *hence greater the pathological changes lower the potency required.*
4. An individual exhibits maximum susceptibility to the simillimum, hence greater the similarity greater is the patient's

Fundamentals of Potency Selection

susceptibility or the ability to get affected in the same plane and thus greater is the potency required.

5. When the remedy is prescribed on poor indications, it resembles poorly with the patient's totality and hence lesser is the patient's susceptibility to it and thus lower is the potency required.

6. A patient lacks susceptibility to a remedy when the remedy is totally out of tune with the patient's totality and hence it would fail to evoke any response in whatever potency it is employed.

POTENCY TYPES IN CENTESIMAL SCALE

The potencies in centesimal scale below the 30th centesimal are termed as low potencies. While 30th centesimal is the lower medium potency and 200th centesimal categorized as the medium potency. All the potencies in the centesimal scale, commencing with 1000 belong to the category of high potencies.

SCIENTIFIC BASIS OF POTENCY SELECTION

A physician has to accurately evaluate every patient's individual susceptibility for selection of potency that matches with the degree of patient's individual susceptibility. Naturally, a blunder in susceptibility assessment would lead to selection of wrong potency. Such improper selection of potency is unscientific. Improper potency selection is reflected in the form of either a poor response or an exaggerated response although the remedy is right. We know that susceptibility varies from individual to individual. This variability of susceptibility is on account of the modification of susceptibility in every individual case which is due to multiple factors which influence the individual susceptibility at a given point of time. A physician is in a position to correctly evaluate individual susceptibility in a given case only if he knows the modifiers of susceptibility. Potency selection on scientific basis requires the physician to examine various factors that modify susceptibility in each case for correct assessment of the degree of patient's susceptibility.

> **INDICATORS OF (DEGREE OF) SUSCEPTIBILITY :**
> - Sensitivity
> - Constitution
> - Past history
> - Type of symptoms
> - Nature of pathology
> - Onset of disease
> - Age
> - Sex
> - Occupation
> - Degree of similarity
> - Nature of selected remedy

The factors that modify susceptibility or are responsible for variability of susceptibility in general are as follows:

1. ONSET OF DISEASE

It is observed that in acute diseases susceptibility is high and in chronic diseases it is low. This statement is true in majority of cases but there are exceptions; sometimes the susceptibility can be low even in acute diseases and high in chronic diseases. For example, in measles without eruptions susceptibility is low. In a chronic case if the degree of similarity of the patient's totality and the remedy is high the patient exhibits increased susceptibility to such a remedy and hence a higher potency can be used.

We can say that diseases characterized by diminished vital action require the low potencies, while diseases characterized by increased vital action respond better to high potencies.

Fundamentals of Potency Selection

2. NATURE OF PATHOLOGY

With the increase in pathological changes in the case there is usually a decrease in the characteristics. Therefore, in cases with advanced pathological changes, disease symptoms predominate. As the individualizing symptoms are very scanty there is diminished susceptibility to remedy. The remedy therefore in such cases is selected on poor indications and susceptibility being low the high potencies can produce 'Killer' type of homeopathic aggravation and hence are contraindicated in such cases.

3. TYPE OF SYMPTOMS

It is observed that provings of low potencies & tinctures produce only more common and general symptoms of the drug which are insufficient to differentiate it from other drugs of the same class. Whereas the finer and more characteristic symptoms of the drug are produced in provings of higher potencies.

Therefore, if the case has finer, peculiar and characteristic symptoms of the selected remedy, the patient's susceptibility to such a remedy is high and hence higher potencies can be used. Similarly cases with predominant mental symptomatology show high degree of susceptibility to rightly selected remedy and here also remedy acts better if employed in higher potency. Closer the similarity of the remedy to the mentals in the case higher is the potency required.

4. NATURE OF SELECTED REMEDY

Susceptibility to organ remedies which are employed for particular effects in definite sphere is low, because such remedies are improperly proved and the required level of clarity of indications for their use is lacking so they are usually selected on poor indications and hence it is better to employ them in lower range of potencies. Similarly the remedies in Biochemic practice are generally administered on coarse indications and hence are usually employed in lower range in decimal scale. However, when selected on finer characteristics, higher range of potencies can be used. Remedies that are inert in crude state show better results in higher potencies.

5. CONSTITUTION

Nervous, impulsive, intelligent and sensitive persons have a higher susceptibility and therefore respond better to higher potencies, whereas sluggish individuals, who are dull of comprehension, idiots and imbeciles, deaf and dumb require low potencies owing to lower susceptibility. *If the patient in question is hypersensitive in general then he will be hypersensitive to homeopathic remedy also hence contrary to the rule that higher the susceptibility higher is the potency employed, in such patients it is better to employ medium and low potencies to be on safer side.*

6. AGE

Susceptibility varies with age. It is higher in infants, children, and young persons. Children are particularly more sensitive during development. Thus, younger people respond to higher potencies better while the older people show better results with lower range of potencies. This does not mean that every infant or child should be given higher potencies and every old man needs low potencies; other factors that differ in every case also need to be taken into consideration prior to arriving at a judgement with regards to patient's susceptibility and the potency required.

7. SEX

Susceptibility is higher in males and males can bear higher potency better. It is lower in females. But during pregnancy it is high while during menses it is low.

8. OCCUPATION

An individual whose job requires much sedentary, intellectual occupation has an increased susceptibility and therefore such individuals are better adapted to higher potencies. Whereas people who are accustomed to long and severe labour outdoors and those who sleep little due to the nature of their occupation (i.e. security guards, labourers etc.) and those in whom the food intake is less are less susceptible and hence better suited to lower potencies. Individuals working in chemical factories, distilleries, and tobacco product manufacturing units or tobacco traders are continuously exposed to chemicals and hence often possess a diminished susceptibility to medicines and thus usually require low potencies. In case their complaints are caused due to allergy to some particular chemical or drug they respond dramatically well to the same chemical or drug given in high potencies.

9. PAST HISTORY

At times the history of past treatments can indicate the type of susceptibility expected in an individual. In mixed up cases, where the patient approaches the physician after lot of allopathic drugging the susceptibility is usually low. Especially when there is history of injudicious homeopathic prescribing due to self-medication or ignorance on part of the homeopathic physician, the susceptibility to the remedy is low and it is better to give low potencies. Similarly in patients who were addicted to narcotic drugs or certain allopathic tablets such as sedatives and laxatives in the recent past or at the time of approaching the physician, the susceptibility is on lower side, hence lower potencies are required. But, Stuart Close states an exception to this rule. He says that in persons having history of taking crude drugs from allopathic and homeopathic "bargain-counter" the susceptibility to crude drugs and low potencies is exhausted and even massive doses have no effect. Such cases respond at once to high potencies of indicated remedy. He concludes by saying that, "the high potency is effective because it acts on virgin soil, invades new territory, as it were."

It should be clear from the above discussion that correct judgement of individual susceptibility is indispensable for choice of right potency. It is not a matter of opinion, as some ignorant clinicians still believe. Solution to the question of potency selection lies in clear understanding of the concept of susceptibility and its relationship with potency, which has been attempted here. Based on these facts some laws of potency selection have been formulated in the above investigation of the concept of susceptibility. Even though the assessment of individual susceptibility is quite difficult when it comes to practice, but having knowledge of factors, which modify the susceptibility and are responsible for its variability in each case is important. It gives a physician some indicators or guideposts in evaluating the individual susceptibility. Thus, facilitating the choice of potency on scientific basis.

∎

CHAPTER 14

Skills of Successful Case Management

- ❖ Remedy Administration — 295
- ❖ Dietary Recommendations — 299
- ❖ Repetition Strategy — 301
- ❖ Scheduling Follow-ups — 303
- ❖ Follow-up Prescription — 304
- ❖ Placebo Prescribing — 313

CHAPTER 14

SKILLS OF SUCCESSFUL CASE MANAGEMENT

A physician's job does not end up with the selection of the homeopathically suitable remedy. On the contrary, it begins after he has selected the medicine to be prescribed. Good prescription is only the first part of case management. What steps are to be taken when the patient reports after first prescription need to be planned in advance. This is known as programming of treatment. Unless it is done we cannot expect the case to reach the desired end. Besides remedy and potency selection other issues like time of administration of medicine, repetition of doses, second prescription and prescribing an intercurrent remedy need to be well thought out and planned for successful case management. Successful case management demands close and unprejudiced observation, right interpretation of patient's report, and ability to have patience when the case shows no signs of improvement. It also requires great courage on part of the treating physician when faced with a difficult situation. Case management for a homeopath is more difficult task as compared to his 'allopathic' colleagues.

> **WHAT IS HOMEOPATHIC CASE MANAGEMENT?**
>
> Homeopathic case management can be defined as a logical and thoughtful selection from among the future courses of action those actions or steps which are necessary to be taken to help the patient reach the desired end (i.e. cure) after the first prescription is made.
>
> It involves unprejudiced observation, logical decision making, planning, programming and implementing what is planned.
>
> Detailed case taking and first prescription is only a beginning of homeopathic case management.

With the accumulation of clinical experience over a period of time it becomes easier for him but the complexities involved still exist due to the great variety of cases he comes across everyday. Dr. M.L. Dhawale rightly describes it as "Razor's edge walk through the amazing territory of remedy response." He further states that, "as the patient progresses under our care the operation cure reveals a changing landscape defined so well by Hering, but little understood by most us." "We never seem to know enough!" Any error in judgement on the part of the treating physician in this important aspect of homeopathic practice can ruin the case even if the remedy is perfectly suitable for the case. Inspite of this, case management still remains the most unattended area in homeopathic education. A student-physician may know how to repertorize a case and how to select a remedy but he seldom knows basics of case management. In practice he finds himself totally helpless when he gets an unfavourable response when the patient reports after the first prescription. Casual follow-up prescriptions worsen the situation further, adding to his difficulties. But in homeopathy no rigid rules can be made regarding what needs to be done when the patient reports for the second time. However, it is possible to formulate some general guidelines regarding case management and follow-ups. Men like Dr. Kent through years of experience and

Skills of Successful Case Management

keen observation of remedy response, have provided some fundamental concepts to homeopathy regarding case management and follow-ups, which prove helpful if understood clearly.

Giving a thorough consideration to following issues is necessary for successful case-management:

1. Remedy Administration
2. Dietary Recommendations
3. Repetition Strategy
4. Scheduling Follow-ups
5. Follow-up Prescription
6. Placebo Prescribing

Let us investigate each one in detail.

1. REMEDY ADMINISTRATION

Remedy administration involves three main factors:

(a) Managing remedy stock
(b) Method of remedy administration
(c) Time of remedy administration

(a) MANAGING REMEDY STOCK

As a general rule a homeopath must keep his set of medicines at a place where they are not directly exposed to direct sunlight, excess heat or cold, moisture and strong odours. He should also advice the patient to take the same precaution while storing medicines at home. Such physical exposures have the ability to destroy the potency of a remedy. We seldom find any directions regarding the period of expiry of homeopathic medicines; as a result individual homeopaths have varying opinions about it, while some of them medicate globules too frequently, others do not feel the need for it even after 1 or 2 years since the time they were first medicated. Globules, especially of those medicines, which are rarely used, turn yellow or brown generally after a period of 1 or 2 years. Various practitioners agree that a change in colour of globules to yellow or brown suggests that it is time to prepare a fresh bottle of medicated globules of the remedy.

In a busy practice it sometimes happens that a physician finds the remedy bottle empty and the remedy dilution exhausted when he badly needs the remedy for a particular patient. In such a situation he should avoid prescribing a substitute in his eagerness to provide medicine to the patient. A homeopath should guard against such hasty prescription of substitute, because in homeopathy there are no substitutes, Bryonia is Bryonia and Rhus tox, is Rhus tox. He should form the habit of checking his stock of medicines periodically to avoid this kind of wrong practice. It is advisable to keep a diary to take note of medicines which are exhausted and for which provision is to be made. A homeopath should have every remedy in at least three potencies so that he can use the right potency when needed. For a beginner, it is advisable to keep every remedy in 30, 200 and 1M potencies of each remedy to start with.

(b) METHOD OF REMEDY ADMINISTRATION

Usually the homeopathic medicines are administered in the form of medicated globules, which are allowed to dissolve on the tongue by mixing with saliva. They may be swallowed as well. The size of globules is physician's choice but greater the size of globules lesser is the number of globules to be given in one dose. *Some physicians are in the habit of directly putting few drops of remedy dilution on patients tongue considering it to be 'more powerful' but administration of medicine through medicated globules is more scientific method of remedy administration as it facilitates better and quick absorption of the remedy.* Crushing a few medicated globules in sugar of milk is also a better method of administering the dose of remedy as the possibility of swallowing the globules without dissolving properly on tongue by the patient is eliminated.

George Vitholkus states, "The homeopath must train himself or herself to pause a moment prior to opening a remedy vial in order to be attentive to any odours in the environment, also it is important that the patient not be wearing any perfume at the time of its administration." Many experienced homeopaths agree that mouth should be free from strong odours while taking the remedy dose, because the presence of strong odours nullifies the effect of remedy. To avoid this a physician should advice every patient to avoid eating or drinking anything, 15 minutes before or after taking the dose. It is best to administer the remedy by dissolving few globules in water when frequent repetition is required. For this few medicated globules crushed in sugar of milk are given to the patient with the advice to dissolve this powder in a small quantity of water and to stir the medicated water every time before taking the dose. One teaspoonful at a time with the interval of 1, 2, 3 or 6 hours depending upon the nature and intensity of complaints is found suitable method of remedy administration.

"Besides the tongue, mouth and stomach which are most commonly affected by the administration of medicine, the nose and respiratory organs are receptive of the action of medicines in fluid form by means of olfaction and inhalation through the mouth," says Hahnemann in paragraph 284 of Organon of Medicine, while describing new ways of remedy administration. In the footnote to the same aphorism he states that in infants medicines act well when administered through the milk of mother or wet nurse. Rubbing the medicine externally which is given internally on back and extremities in cases of old diseases is another mode of remedy administration described by Hahnemann in paragraph 285 of Organon of Medicine.

(c) TIME OF REMEDY ADMINISTRATION

Apart from method of administration the time of remedy administration is also equally important for good case management. A dose at (especially of constitutional remedy) bedtime is best in chronic cases as during sleep, there is repose of mind and body, which creates right kind of conditions for the action of homeopathic remedy. When the remedy is to be prescribed in repeated doses throughout the day, the morning dose should be taken before breakfast and before brushing the teeth to avoid presence of strong odours in mouth at the time of taking the remedy. Especially Sulphur is best given on an empty stomach in the morning as it may produce insomnia if given at night to a patient not having insomnia.

According to Clarke the reverse is true for Arsenic iod. It should be given preferably after meals to avoid distressing stomach symptoms.

Another precaution with regards to time of administration of remedies is to avoid administering either before or during the time of aggravation of the remedy. It is better to give a remedy after the period of aggravation is over. For example, Arsenicum album should not be administered at midday or midnight, whereas it is advisable to avoid administering Colocynth, Lycopodium, and Helleborous in evening especially between 4 to 8 pm and Natrium mur. should not be given in morning and likewise others depending on their time of aggravation.

In chronic cases, worst time to administer a constitutional remedy is during acute exacerbation of the chronic disease. The acute exacerbation should be controlled by a related acute or short acting remedy which prepares the ground for constitutional remedy to be followed afterwards. While prescribing for menstrual troubles of long standing, it is better to administer the constitutional remedy after menses rather than during menses. Similarly, in asthma cases the constitutional remedy should be administered after every attack and never during attack. According to Dr. Dhawale longer periods of remission before final disappearance of symptoms are observed in cases treated in such manner. In diseases characterized by periodicity, a deep acting remedy should not be administered just before or during a paroxysm. In a case of malaria, failure to take this precaution is known to have precipitated severe paroxysms of malaria which can prove fatal especially in case of infants.

2. DIETARY RECOMMENDATIONS

Irregularities in diet can serve as a major obstacle in the recovery process, hence it goes without saying that a homeopath must advice the type of diet to be taken during treatment. Dietary recommendations regarding the particular foods to be avoided are also necessary. Dietary restrictions to be suggested depend on the type of disease the patient is suffering from. Thus, a patient of renal calculi should be advised to drink lot of water and to avoid tomatoes and spinach, which can contribute in stone formation owing to the oxalic acid content. While a diabetic is advised to avoid sugar in any form, a patient of bronchitis must be told to strictly avoid smoking. Similarly, a patient of recurrent aphthus stomatitis to totally avoid pungent food, tobacco chewing and eating supari (beetalnut). However, a physician should not impose abrupt stoppage of long accustomed addictions like tea, coffee, tobacco and liquor, etc. The patient should be advised to gradually reduce the intake of such substances as their sudden withdrawal can produce withdrawal symptoms. But if the patient's disease is a result of his addictions, physician has to insist on quick control and total avoidance of such maintaining causes.

Instructions for avoiding the food products which may interfere with action of homeopathic remedy and antidote its effects are equally necessary. Anything having medicinal properties can antidote a remedy. For example, coffee is a medicinal substance that overstimulates the nervous system and coffee being a well known antidote to homeopathic remedies, the patient should be instructed to avoid coffee altogether. Patient may knowingly or unknowingly take some food products having small quantity of coffee but that should not bother a physician. It is not advisable to take any 'allopathic drugs' during homeopathic treatment especially sedatives and steroids, etc. except in terminally ill patients who cannot survive without these drugs. Antihypertensive drugs and drugs related to heart ailments should not be withdrawn suddenly and a thorough knowledge of patient's condition is necessary before the patient is advised to stop them. But, as a general rule, the patient should be instructed to avoid any over-the-counter drugs and self medication as this may change the symptom picture making it impossible to find out which medicine produced results, and thus making it difficult to make a second prescription. Camphor too antidotes homeopathic remedies, usually vapo-rubs and inhalers used for common cold contain camphor and should be avoided. Things having strong aromatic odours such as clove oil, raw onions and garlic are also contraindicated for homeopathic patient. Mint in toothpaste has been known to antidote homeopathic remedies although such cases are very rare. Normal intake of common food items seems to have no medicinal effects and hence do not interfere with the action of homeopathic remedy.

> **In this connection there is a wise rule:**
> " Chronic cases should not eat to excess of that which they especially crave, whereas Acute patients may and should eat largely of what they crave, if the craving comes on with the illness."
>
> **— Elizabeth Wright-Hubbard, MD**

We find mention of particular foods causing and aggravating the complaints in certain remedies in materia medica. Therefore, a patient also needs to be instructed regarding the foods to be avoided depending on the remedy that is prescribed to him. For example, a patient under the action of Pulsatilla should be advised to avoid fatty food such as 'ghee,' oil, eggs, etc. Whereas the one taking Argentum nitricum should be told to avoid sweets and candy. Similarly, when Nux vomica is prescribed, the patient should be instructed to avoid tobacco, beer, alcohol and other stimulants. A reference to the rubric "food agg." or "disordered by" in repertory can serve as a guide to the physician regarding such type of dietary recommendations. Physician and family members of the patient should not put strict restrictions on patients with acute disease, when there is strong craving for certain foods in such patients, as such hindrances in the gratification of the desire can oppose the radical removal of the disease, states Hahnemann in paragraph 259 to 263 of Organon of Medicine which prove beneficial when put to practice. R. E. Dudgeon describes the essence of dietary recommendations by saying, *"Our dietetic rules must be adapted, like our medicinal prescriptions, to each individual case."*

3. REPETITION STRATEGY

Injudicious repetition of a remedy is the major cause of failure in homeopathic case management. Accuracy in judgement in this area is much more necessary than in any other operation of homeopathic practice. One must know the general criteria for repetition enumerated or laid down by homeopathic masters.

The criteria for repetition are as follows:
(a) No repetition is necessary once an adequate response is noticed.
(b) No further repetition, as long as the good response continues.
(c) Cessation of progress should not be taken as an indication for repetition.

(d) Repetition necessary when the symptoms that have disappeared under the action of remedy return.

In acute cases with severe intensity of complaints, repetition at intervals of few hours is necessary especially in cases of fever. Repetition should be stopped as soon as the response is visible. It is better to gradually reduce the repetition. Premature cessation of remedy is known to promote a relapse. Usually, for frequent repetitions the medicine is given in water, and the patient is advised to stop taking it as soon as the amelioration is observed. In acute cases where the symptoms are of moderate severity the remedy can be repeated twice, thrice daily for 3 to 4 days, depending upon the type of complaints and the severity of complaints.

All the masters agree that as a general rule in chronic cases it is best to give only a single dose and then wait for a period of at least 10 to 15 days. The action of single dose may continue for one or at times two months. But if assessment of response after 10 to 15 days reveals that the remedy was right still there is no change and that single dose stimulation was insufficient another does may be given. In our eagerness to cure, it is commonly assumed that, a second dose of good remedy will speed up the case but here lies our greatest error. Sometimes the physician, in a hurry, is tempted to repeat a dose even when the patient reports amelioration with some minor symptoms still persisting, 'to complete the cure' but it is the greatest blunder one can commit in homeopathic case management.

Reappearance of symptoms or mere cessation of progress is not an indication for repetition of dose. Only when the symptoms, which have reappeared, do not disappear of their own accord repetition is required. In cases where the pathological changes have progressed considerably the vitality of the patient is low, and frequent repetitions in such cases often proves dangerous due to the fact that reaction induced by rapidly repeated doses can be too violent for the patient to bear. Considerable degree of patience on part of the treating homeopath is a must, especially in chronic cases. We can conclude that 'Not doing anything' is more important than doing something for successful case management after the first right prescription. Thus, it is a paradox *"The one who repeats least is a better prescriber than the one who repeats often carelessly."*

4. SCHEDULING FOLLOW-UPS

After the treatment of the patient has begun, review of the patient's condition after a certain period becomes necessary to know the progress made by the patient. As such, it is essential that the next appointment with the patient should be fixed in the first meeting with the patient. Although, the time to evaluate a patient after first visit varies with the nature and type of case in hand, however, certain general recommendations can be proposed. No one needs to be told that in acute cases and severely suffering chronic cases the follow-up visits should be scheduled at shorter intervals, whereas in chronic cases at longer intervals. In severely suffering acute patients time for follow-up should be few hours after the first prescription. In such cases the patient is told to report at an interval of 6, 8, 12, or 24 hours while in those acute cases where the symptoms are not very intense the patient can be called after an interval of 2, 3, or 4 days depending on the nature of case. Patient in general should be advised to report immediately if there are any dramatic changes requiring attention of the physician after first prescription. In such an event patient should be advised not to wait for the doses to be consumed.

In chronic cases, the ideal interval is 10 to 15 days after the first prescription. In those cases where there is a possibility of very sluggish response, it is advisable to call the patient after an interval of 1 month or so. Contrary to the popular belief, evaluation of patients on week-to-week basis is best to be avoided in chronic cases because such frequent visits do not only put undue pressure on the physician to 'do something' but it is inconvenient for the patient also to report at short intervals. Due to pressure from the patient the physician may fall prey to prescribing "in between" when it is time to wait and watch. This often proves damaging to the case. Thus, by keeping longer intervals between follow-ups it is possible for the physician to keep off pressure and avoid erroneous "in between" prescribing and consequent failures.

Acute Cases	Follow up Schedule
• Severely suffering patients.	6, 8, 12, or 24 hours.
• Patients with symptoms of moderate intensity.	Review after 2, 3, or 4 days.
Note: In acute cases the patient should be advised to report immediately if there are any dramatic changes needing attention of the physician.	
Chronic Cases	**Follow up Schedule**
• Cases where quick response is expected.	8 to 10 days.
• Cases where a tardy response seems likely (considering the nature of disease and susceptibility of the patient).	15 to 20 days. (week to week evaluation avoided).
• Chronic cases with possibility of very sluggish response.	One month.

5. FOLLOW-UP PRESCRIPTION

Follow-up prescription is more important than first prescription because homeopathic failures often result from faulty follow-up prescription. A wrong follow-up prescription spoils the case or at least makes the case very difficult to cure. Errors in second prescription result from either inaccuracy in recording patient's responses or misinterpretation of the responses. Let us investigate these two factors in detail:

(a) RECORDING PATIENT'S RESPONSES

There are two aspects of recording patient's responses — the first, what should be recorded? and the second How to record it? Majority of the homeopaths are in the habit of noting down responses in too simple terms such as 'complaints >' or 'complaints <' or 'complaints remain unchanged.' Instead of general remarks like these it is better to inquire into each symptom and record the changes in each symptom. Inquiry and recording of appearance of any new symptoms, which were not there before the first prescription is also necessary. Apart from specific information regarding each symptom the patient needs to be asked how does he or she feels in general. In some cases recording of changes occurring on the mental or emotional plane after the first prescription is also necessary in the follow-up interview. The golden rule is the same as that in case taking, let the patient speak and elaborate without cutting his description in the middle. Physician should restrain from asking questions according to his own format of recording the follow-up responses when the patient is describing the changes after the first prescription. Once the patient completes his / her description, the physician should ask information relevant to his requirements. This is most important for accurate recording of responses. It is best to start the follow-up inquiry with some general question like 'How are you?'

The second question i.e. 'How to record responses?' may be answered by saying that note down whatever the patient tells. However the answer is not that simple; judgment with regards to the reliability of responses is also necessary. Mechanical recording without giving consideration to the reliability of what is said may lead to erroneous second prescription. It is a mistake to assume that whatever the patient informs might have actually occurred to the patient after the first prescription. But it is important to analyse patient's responses before putting them on paper. While trusting the patient it is also necessary to scrutinize the information provided by the patient. This is because two patients may not respond to first prescription in the same manner although the degree of amelioration due to first prescription in both the cases may be the same. There must always be variation in the manner in which two patients report after first prescription. The response that a physician receives after first prescription is not entirely dependent upon the accuracy of the first prescription or the remedy given but greatly on the individual patient who is responding. Keen observation of the patient's body language and the manner in which he describes the effect of first prescription, often reveal to the physician the difference between, 'what it appears to be' and 'what it actually is.' A patient who is not sure of the physician's ability to treat and cure him or who is a non-believer in homeopathy may give a report which would lead the physician to think that the remedy has failed to act. Such patients usually ignore to report precise or trivial changes or slight improvement in their condition due to their personal prejudices about the physician and the science or due to the belief that any positive report may divest physician's attention to their treatment. Whereas an overzealous patient, who is a firm believer in homeopathy with unfathomable faith in physician's ability, may give an exaggerated version of improvement of his condition. Whereas an oversensitive patient with fear of so called 'Homeopathic aggravations' may report an aggravation of his complaints even when the first prescription he received was a placebo. Major obstacle in accurate recording of response is created when the patient sends any of his family members to report and to 'bring the medicine.' Whatever may be the reason for it but in such a case, physician does not find himself in a position to take stock of the actual situation. The representative of the patient often

Skills of Successful Case Management

gives an altered version of patients condition or uses vague terms like 'he/she is worst' or 'he/she is better' to describe the patient's condition. As the correct assessment of patient's condition is not possible, such practice should not be encouraged. The physician should insist on patient's presence in the follow-up visit. This may not be always possible in case of outstation patients. In such cases the patient should be advised to have telephonic communication with the physician.

Even though, with experience a physician acquires considerable degree of accuracy in analyzing the patient's responses before recording them in the follow-up visit. For a novice keen observation of the manner of description, the knowledge of variability in responses in different individuals together with balance in trusting and suspecting the patients version lead to accuracy in recording of responses in course of practice.

(b) INTERPRETATION OF PATIENT'S RESPONSES

Interpretation of responses means perceiving — What has happened? Why it has happened? and What needs to be done? As far as interpretation of complex responses is concerned, which we might get in the course of homeopathic treatment, experience is the best teacher. The changes in patient's condition after the first prescription are dependent on various factors that influence him during the course of treatment and they vary greatly from case to case and hence there are numerous possibilities. All the possibilities and eventualities during homeopathic treatment cannot be predicted before hand nor can anybody give a clear explanation about every response received during treatment. Case examples often prove insufficient to guide the physician with regards to interpretation of responses in second visit, because the cases described are different from the cases one meets in his own practice and no two cases can ever be alike. However, the responses a homeopath commonly comes across in his day-to-day practice can be discussed.

> **COMMONLY REPORTED RESPONSES AFTER FIRST PRESCRIPTION**
> 1. No Change.
> 2. Amelioration.
> 3. Aggravation.
>   (a) Short and Simple.
>   (b) Severe and Prolonged.
>   (c) Killer type.
>   (d) Medicinal.
> 4. Incomplete Amelioration or Arrested Progress.

Each response needs to be investigated and assessed logically to decide future course of action.

(i) No Change

In an acute case no change in patient's symptoms suggests that the remedy selected was wrong. In such a situation the possible interpretation is that the remedy first prescribed was least similar to the case. However, if on re-examination of the case it is observed that the remedy closely resembles the patient's totality it means that either the potency was not suitable or the repetitions were insufficient. Whereas in a chronic case if there is no change in the patient's symptoms it does not mean that the remedy was wrong, because if a deep acting constitutional remedy is prescribed in a chronic case it may take weeks or sometimes even month or two before a patient reports a change. So here it is a time to wait and placebo must be prescribed. But when there is no change even after lapse of reasonable period then it indicates that the case needs to be reviewed and re-examined to find a more suitable remedy.

(ii) Amelioration

When the patient reports amelioration without even a slight aggravation, the physician can be sure that the remedy and potency

Skills of Successful Case Management

both are right. It also indicates a good prognosis for the patient. In this situation no repetition of the remedy is necessary till the symptoms return in full swing again. When the patient reports amelioration the best prescription is therefore placebo. But the time taken for amelioration after taking the first dose and the sequence of disappearance of symptoms must be inquired.

(iii) Aggravation

Aggravation of the symptoms is the least desirable response for the physician as well as the patient. Especially for the beginner it is a panic situation. He is most likely to commit mistakes in the case management and future course of prescribing when patient reports back with aggravated symptoms. While an ignorant physician will try to pacify the patient by reassuring him that it is a good sign in homeopathic treatment. However, both are at fault. When the patient reports aggravation it is neither a time to get frightened unnecessarily nor a time to rejoice thinking it to be a 'good sign.' A homeopath must see the aggravation in the right perspective. Interpretation of aggravation is much more difficult than interpretation of any other response. Mistakes in interpretation of aggravation are common due to the fact that misconceptions about aggravation exist in large majority of practitioners and even in qualified homeopaths. Contrary to the popular belief, aggravation by no means is an essential part of the treatment. The ideal of cure in homeopathy is 'rapid gentle and permanent and in most harmless way' — we can't forget that. A good prescriber rarely comes across aggravation in his practice. Errors result from conveniently considering it a 'good omen.' Before considering it either good or bad it is important to perceive what type of aggravation it is. Aggravation resulting after administration of homeopathic remedy can be of four varieties:

- Short and simple aggravation.
- Severe and prolonged aggravation.

- Killer type of aggravation
- Medicinal aggravation.

Short and Simple Aggravation: A short and simple aggravation followed by amelioration of complaints is good and indicates that the remedy was accurately selected. In this type of aggravation no new symptoms are noticed. It also means that organic changes are not advanced. This type of aggravation should not be interfered by the physician. Only placebo is necessary in such a situation.

Severe & Prolonged Aggravation: Never commit the mistake of considering a severe and prolonged aggravation as a bad omen, because a patient having such type of aggravation when observed for some time, reports a slow improvement and gradual amelioration of symptoms although the initial response was an aggravation and it continued for some time. It means that the remedy was right and the prognosis is good. One may have a question that if the remedy was right then what was responsible for severe and prolonged aggravation. This may be because the disease was in advanced stage, the vitality was low, and there were structural changes. The case could have become incurable if the remedy would have been wrong. It was a borderline case. The other possible reason for this type of response is the inaccuracy in potency selection. The potency may have been higher than required. It is difficult to distinguish this type of aggravation from the killer type of aggravation and medicinal aggravation.

'Killer' Type Aggravation: This type of aggravation is seen in incurable cases with gross pathological changes in vital organs. It usually results from prescribing a deep-acting constitutional remedy in high potency. It is better to prescribe a similar superficially acting remedy in low potency for palliation. An over enthusiastic and ignorant physician who presumes that homeopathy can cure everything under the sky often falls in the trap of this type of 'Killer' aggravation. Whereas the one who knows the value of diagnosis in homeopathic practice and the importance of selecting cases before treating them rarely comes across such unwanted situation.

Medicinal Aggravation: Hahnemann writes about this worst type of aggravation in paragraph 249 and its footnote in Organon of Medicine. In this type of aggravation the patient reports that the original symptoms remain as it is and in addition to it new symptoms have appeared. It indicates that the remedy selection was wrong and remedy is probably proving itself. If the remedy is neither deep-acting nor given in high potency, this type of aggravation will go off on its own after sometime. But if the aggravation becomes serious and persists inspite of waiting, immediate administration of a new remedy by taking into consideration both new and old symptoms is required. Sometimes the oversensitive and idiosyncratic patients develop some symptoms of the remedy especially when the potency is inappropriate although the remedy is right because 'some patients prove every remedy they get.' In such cases the remedy symptoms usually pass of automatically after sometime followed by improvement in patient's condition.

(iv) Incomplete Amelioration or Arrested Progress

Sometimes a patient reports amelioration of complaints after first prescription but the amelioration does not last long or the remedy first prescribed gives considerable relief but no further progress is witnessed. The possible interpretation of this response is that although the remedy was right, it might have been antidoted. This type of response is seen when the patient does something with or without knowledge that cuts short the action of the remedy. He might take coffee, alcohol or tobacco or there is possibility that he might have come in contact with substance that antidotes homeopathic remedy. If the relapse of symptoms presents exactly the same picture, the same remedy in same potency is needed. The other reason for this type of response is that although the remedy was right the potency might have been too low. A re-examination of the case might indicate that the chronic illness has already progressed to structural changes in organs.

Sometimes the remedy and potency both seem to be right but still the patient is not completely relieved or there is considerable relief but no further progress. The question here is how to change the remedy or potency when both are right? The arrested progress in such case is due to the fact that the selected remedy has done all the good work it could do and a remedy that bears a complementary relation to the preceding one is required. This complementary remedy when administered would complete the action of first one. For example in a case of recurrent tonsillitis Belladonna is indicated in acute phase while its complementary Calc. carb. might be required to complete its action, as it is a deep acting remedy to complete the curative process. Whereas Nat. mur. which is a chronic of Ignatia might be required in a case where Ignatia was first prescribed and ameliorated the patient to considerable degree.

In chronic case one may find that the case comes to standstill and even after administration of well-selected constitutional remedy, there is no further progress. In such a situation a re-study of the case to find out the dominant miasm responsible for arrested progress is necessary. The suitable anti-miasmatic remedy needs to be administered to remove the 'block' so that, when the constitutional remedy is administered, the case begins to progress and a better response follows.

(v) Amelioration Followed by Aggravation

Amelioration followed by severe aggravation indicates a bad prognosis. This type of response is usually seen in incurable cases. Here only palliation is possible and a new remedy should be selected after restudying the case. The other reason for such response is the faulty remedy selection. It results from the fact that the selected remedy was superficially similar and hence a new remedy is required.

> **Remember your cardinal principles:**
>
> - Never repeat a remedy when the patient himself is improving.
> - Never change a remedy when the symptoms are following Hering's Law of Cure in the reverse order of symptoms.
> - Never change your remedy when a discharge or eruption follows the administration.
>
> — Elizabeth Wright-Hubbard

6. PLACEBO PRESCRIBING

Placebo means a medicine like substance administered to gratify a patient or a pharmacologically inactive substance administered as a drug that is known to have a psychological effect on the patient. It is the most useful instrument or tool in homeopathic case management. Placebo is like a blessing for a wise physician when facing a complex situation in case management. For a patient it is 'blessing in disguise.' Staurt Close rightly calls it as the 'Second best remedy.'

Placebo has numerous uses in homeopathic practice. It is the best medicine to start the treatment of a chronic case when the physician is not certain about the suitable remedy for the case. By prescribing placebo physician gets the much-needed time to study the case and select the appropriate remedy. At times the patient's response after the first prescription makes it necessary to observe the patient for few more days without prescribing anything. In such 'wait and watch' situation placebo is physician's best friend. Here it satisfies the patient's need for continued medication and at the same time, gives the physician a chance to observe and interpret 'what is happening.' For anxious patients placebo is the best support. The psychological effect of placebo is quiet surprising. It has proved effective in people of all ages and widely differing levels of intelligence. The most wonderful fact with regards to use of placebo is that the physician who is using it is sure that he is doing no harm to his patient.

Stuart Close very correctly described it as a 'trade secret' worth millions. This is true today than it was ever before, because the number of people taking homeopathic treatment is rapidly and continuously increasing throughout the world. There is growing awareness about homeopathy and its effectiveness in treating various diseases. As a result, the present day patient is well informed before he visits a homeopathic clinic. There is every chance that he knows that homeopaths prescribe placebo at times. But a homeopath cannot imagine case management without placebo and hence the placebo must be 'well disguised.' The best possible way to make the placebo look and feel like medicine is by using globules medicated with some plain alcohol or dispensing alcohol. A licence to store and use alcohol might be necessary. It depends on the laws of the region where one is practicing. If the licence is must then the concerned physician must obtain it. Elizabeth Wright Hubbard has given a very useful tip regarding use of placebo. She states, "It is nice to train the patients to take powders or pellets as placebo which are similar in appearance to the actual remedies, and not to give them the tempting brown, pink and green blank tablets."

A physician has to take many precautions while dispensing placebo. The first is that it should be the physician's most closely guarded secret. No one except the physician himself should know that he is using placebo. He should never admit its use in private or in public. The placebo bottles must be filled when necessary by the physician himself behind closed doors. He should never inform

Skills of Successful Case Management

his assistant staff regarding the single dose and use of blank doses. A way to keep the placebo 'visible but hidden' is by making two medicine cabinets, one containing genuine medicine bottles and the other containing neatly labelled bottles of blank globules. As far as the naming of placebo bottles is concerned it is a physician's choice. But it is better to have names resembling those of homeopathic medicines like, 'Phytum' 'Phillinum' or 'Nihilinum' etc. One way is to label the bottles in the placebo cabinet from Aconitum to Zincum with some special sign to indicate that the bottle contains placebo. For example, the bottle in the genuine medicine cabinet is labelled as 'Aconite 30' while that in placebo cabinet is labelled as 'Aconite 30c.'

Apart from globules moistened with alcohol, plain globules crushed in sugar of milk or plain sugar tablets or diskettes can be used as a placebo. A physician should never think that by using placebo he is fooling his patients. Hahnemann once said that a physician should have the character enough to prescribe a placebo when indicated. He has referred to it as a 'divine gift of god.'

CHAPTER 15

The 20 Don'ts of Homeopathic Practice

CHAPTER 5

The 70 Points of Homeopathic Practice

CHAPTER 15

THE 20 DON'TS OF HOMEOPATHIC PRACTICE

The very nature of homeopathy demands great caution on part of the treating physician, hence it becomes more important to know what should not be done in homeopathic practice rather than knowing what should be done. Some general suggestions with regards to the don'ts of homeopathic practice are as follows:

1. **Don't try to treat every patient that seeks your treatment.** Remember, homeopathy can do miracles only in cases which fall within the scope of the science. Due care in selection of cases is the first step towards successful homeopathic practice.

2. **Don't make false promises; neither assure great results to a patient when the case falls out of the limitations of homeopathy and your own limitations.** Your assurances regarding the extent of relief you can offer him should be based on clear consideration of the type of complaints, nature, intensity & chronicity of disease in his case.

3. **Don't be rude and irritated while communicating with the patient even if he is not co-operating.** Instead try to convince him and make him understand how important it is to get

detailed information before treatment. A rude behaviour always serves as the greatest obstacle in establishing rapport with the patient essential for good case taking.

4. **Don't avoid physical examination considering it to be of secondary importance for a homeopath.** Also don't hesitate to advice laboratory investigations where necessary.

5. **Don't avoid detailed case taking, considering it time consuming, laborious and difficult.** It is the first step to cure and not a formality. Remember, 'No pains no gains.'

6. **Don't avoid record keeping at all.** A record is the best guide for follow up and management of the case; without it a physician is in total dark when the patient reports for follow up.

7. **Don't put too much emphasis on one or two prominent symptoms of the case or pathological findings in the case while prescribing.** Prescribe for totality and prescribe for the individual and not for the disease he is suffering from.

8. **Don't be in the bad habit of prescribing a drug just by thumbing through favourite repertory.** All of us at one time or the other had the temptation to prescribe the remedy that appears in bold letters in one or two important symptoms of the case. It is best to consult materia medica if you don't have the time to carry out a detailed repertorization.

9. **Don't use a particular repertory every time for repertorization just because it is your favourite repertory.** Let the case decide which repertory it needs.

10. **Don't be casual in symptom to rubric conversion.** The rubric selected must carry the exact meaning of the symptom.

11. **Don't prescribe your favourite remedy every time you see a case of a particular disease.** Remember, diseases may be the same but one who suffers from it has different individuality or totality from the other having the same disease.

12. **Don't avoid prescribing some remedy because of your personal prejudices, prejudices are like termites of prescribing.** Remember, a remedy is neither good or bad for any particular disease condition; if it is homeopathic to the case in hand it will surely prove effective.
13. **Don't prescribe a second remedy before giving a consideration to the type of relationship it has with the one prescribed earlier.** Remember, a remedy having an inimical relationship to the one employed earlier proves damaging to the case.
14. **Don't select a particular potency on personal preferences** and the so-called 'personal experiences'. Let the susceptibility of the patient and the type of case in hand decide the potency needed.
15. **Don't be averse to a particular range of potencies; all are equally effective and prove useful when selected scientifically.**
16. **Don't prescribe when the patient reports amelioration of complaints.** 'The right remedy at wrong time always spoils the case.'
17. **Don't change the remedy unless the symptom picture is clear and you are sure of your choice.**
18. **Don't hesitate to repeat the drug frequently or infrequently considering the type of case in hand and the demands of the case.** Frequent repetition is not always dangerous contrary to the popular belief, sometimes it is necessary.
19. **Don't be overzealous to continue treating a case too long when it is evident that the patient is not showing any sign of improvement and his condition is deteriorating inspite of your best efforts.** One should not hesitate to refer such a case to more experienced & competent physician.

20. **Don't hesitate to refer a book in the presence of the patient, when you find it necessary.** Remember, referring a book neither lowers your dignity, nor puts a question mark on your knowledge.

CHAPTER 16

Clinical Training in Homeopathic Practice

- ❖ Institute of Clinical Research — 327
- ❖ Athenian School of Homeopathic Medicine — 328
- ❖ Clinical Training Center for Classical Homeopathy — 329
- ❖ Systematic Homoeopathic Practice Orientation and Training Programme (Shot) — 330
- ❖ Homoeopathic Study Circle — 331
- ❖ Dr Robin Murphy, ND — 332
- ❖ Dr Frederik Schroyens, MD — 333
- ❖ Dr Roger van Zandvoort — 334
- ❖ Dr Luc De Schepper, MD — 335
- ❖ Dr Jeremy Sherr — 335

CHAPTER 16

CLINICAL TRAINING IN HOMEOPATHIC PRACTICE

If I were to ask, what should be taught to make a competent homeopath? Most will answer, "The Organon, Materia Medica, Repertory, etc." Unfortunately this is not the correct answer, because homeopathic practice is fundamentally a skill. It is more of a vocation than a traditional knowledge like history, chemistry or biology. So the focus of education should be on imparting skills and more importantly the homeopathic attitude rather than knowing Hahnemann, provings, remedies, etc. The traditional homeopathic education in India involves going through 4 to 5 years of lectures, listening, reading, studying, memorizing and regurgitating the information before having an opportunity to deal with the real situations in practice. As a result the output from this machinery is a homeopath full of homeopathic information but lacking in clinical skills and homeopathic attitude much needed for successful homeopathic practice. As a result, a homeopathic graduate meets with many difficulties when he takes the plunge in homeopathic practice. In spite of all the homeopathic education he has received till graduation, eliciting the story from the patient remains his biggest difficulty. His case record often lacks individuality and at times remains incomplete. The emotional side of the case eludes him till last. He thus has no case at all. The obvious difficulty that follows this is the inability to evolve patient's image, out of the maze of symptoms. Even when he succeeds in evolving patient's image the next step which involves identifying patient's image with a single remedy image from homeopathic materia medica is difficult for him. A fresh graduate lacks confidence in acute prescribing and a chronic case with mixed up symptomatology often confuses him and proves to be a nightmare. If the student-physician tries to seek guidance from a senior practitioner it is difficult to get such a practitioner, as there are very few practitioners who let a student work for a time with them. It usually takes hard work and luck to find a good homeopath to act as a preceptor.

In order to achieve reasonable clinical efficiency, which is must to get results and practice homeopathy scientifically, clinical training in homeopathic practice is the best solution for fresh graduates, who aspire to become skilled and competent homeopaths. It is also suited to those practicing physicians who find it difficult to translate theory into practice. Clinical training can be defined as the type of education in which the learner is guided or trained in the methodology of homeopathic practice, to help him in gaining reasonable clinical efficiency and clinical judgement necessary while handling various cases. The student is given wide clinical exposure so as to make the transition from the more introspective educational experience of the classroom to actual practice of homeopathy. The focus of clinical training is on methodology of practice, which includes case taking, case-analysis, and case management. Here the learning is problem based. It means the problem (i.e. the patient) is encountered first in the learning process, then the students have to evaluate and decide what knowledge and/or skills are needed to solve the problem. This motivates them to study and use appropriate resources. This is a better way of learning because homeopathic practice is intrinsically problem based in nature. The basic problem is "what remedy can I find for this patient?" A clinical training in scientific homeopathy (popularly known as classical homeopathy) teaches the learner to combine the theoretical knowledge of homeopathy with the actual case in hand. It helps the learner/student to stay down to earth when faced with the problem of the patient and also helps to avoid theorizing. It is best suited to those physicians who want to start the study of homeopathy and at the same time want to start treating patients to see results in practice.

A highly motivated student with good therapeutic qualities and talents is sure to get transformed into a competent homeopathic physician, after completion of the type of training provided by clinical training centre. The curriculum in these centres is designed to emphasize the practical application of the art and science of homeopathy along scientific lines. The curriculum mainly includes interviewing techniques, case analysis, symptom interpretation, repertory work, and case related study of materia medica and long-term management of cases. The comprehensive training one receives is a blend of observation and clinical skills.

The details of some of the clinical training centres in India and those around the world are given below, hoping that they would be of help to the one who aspires to receive such training.

1. INSTITUTE OF CLINICAL RESEARCH

The Institute of Clinical Research was established in 1975 by the internationally acclaimed homeopathic clinician, educationist and author, the late Dr. M. L. Dhawale (1927-1987), in response to the need of evolving a scientific and accurate system of homeopathic practice, education and research. It was established with the objective to help student-physicians to become competent homeopaths. This would mean that at the successful conclusion of the course the student would be competent to handle various types of cases in his private practice with confidence. The other objective is to help the student-physicians to achieve clinical judgement through balanced and logical clinical thinking. Graduates or Diploma holders from any of the recognized colleges of medicine (allopathic, homeopathic or ayurvedic) can apply towards the end of their internship. Medical practitioners who can spare time and have interest and the commitment are also eligible for the courses conducted by I.C.R. The duration of the course is minimum three terms of 6 months each. The admissions begin in March and September of each year. The duration is individualized and is discussed in the admission interview. The training involves clinical exposure at various OPD's and IPD's of the I.C.R., the MLD trust and its staff where the student is guided in the science and art of case-taking, recording and processing on the standardized case record. Guided discussion sessions and expositions are held from time to time. Periodic and final evaluation of the student is a regular feature. The course is case-centered and involves interaction with many competent homeopaths and exposure to multiple standardized homeopathic clinics. There is an entrance test comprising of theory and case. Admission interviews are usually held in the third week of March / September. A course on the similar lines is conducted at Pune branch of ICR.

2. ATHENIAN SCHOOL OF HOMEOPATHIC MEDICINE

The Athenian centre was founded by George Vithoulkas in 1970. It is one of the largest homeopathic clinics in the world. This centre offers homeopathic education to doctors and medical students and also functions as a clinic where 30 medical doctors practice homeopathy. The formal introductory course lasts for two years and is open to selected medical doctors and medical students only. The first year concentrates on philosophy, theory, and study of Organon. In the second year, the emphasis is on materia medica, use of the repertory and case analysis. Lectures take place two evenings a week and are conducted in the Greek language. In 1982 a programme was initiated for foreign medical doctors. There are two positions in the clinic that can be taken up by English speaking doctors. This training is for one year and such doctors treat foreign patients living in Athens. The clinic also treats selected foreign patients who come to Athens for regular visits.

On completion of the introductory course the physician-student begins a three-year internship in which he / she has full-time clinical duties examining new patients. These patients then remain under the student's care but during the first year a clinic supervisor reviews each case thoroughly. Through the study of individual cases and further study of materia medica and case analysis the doctor gains proficiency. During the second and third year the doctor is encouraged to take more and more responsibility in making his own homeopathic prescriptions. Homeopathy has been accepted by the Greek government and will be incorporated into the national health system, keeping in view the excellent standard of homeopathy in the Athens clinic.

3. CLINICAL TRAINING CENTER FOR CLASSICAL HOMEOPATHY

Dr. Alfons Geukens founded the clinical training center for classical homeopathy at Hechtel-Eksel Belgium in 1980. Dr. Alfons Geukens is a very popular teacher and orator all over the world. His method of teaching is very practical and down to earth interspersed with homeopathic humor. His training center has quickly grown into a highly respected training center for doctors dedicated to learning classical homeopathy. Dr. Geukens has studied extensively with George Vithoulkas. Every year in

September Dr. Geukens starts a new course in classical homeopathy. The duration of the course is three years. There are lectures on Saturday from 9 am to 5pm. The trainee has to follow a supervision of 150 hours besides the Saturday lecturers. Apart from Dr. Alfons Geukens there are four other supervisors in the center they are Dr.Guido Mortelmans, Dr.Henk Van Hootegem, Dr. Kris Gaublomne, and Dr. Fons Vanden Berghe. In the three year programme the doctor-trainee must attend the lectures given by Dr. Geukens in the Netherlands. The trainee begins by taking the homeopathic case and then discusses the patient with one of the supervisors. The trainee together with the supervisor decides on the remedy to be given.

4. SYSTEMATIC HOMOEOPATHIC PRACTICE ORIENTATION AND TRAINING PROGRAMME (SHOT)

'SHOT' or Systematic Homoeopathic practice Orientation and Training programme is a certificate course in Central India (Nagpur, Maharashtra) and the first of its kind. Dr Anurag Deshmukh developed this programme aimed at giving practical training to budding homeopaths, in the year 2005. 'SHOT' is an orientation programme that aims at transforming a student from just being a homeopathic graduate to a confident homeopathic physician. It is specially designed for interns, fresh homeopathic graduates, postgraduate students and budding homeopaths. It is also suited for those practicing homeopaths who want to achieve excellence in homeopathic practice because it is most helpful in building confidence in clinical practice. It can help the already practicing physicians in achieving clinical judgement through unprejudiced thinking.

Student physicians have a million questions about homeopathic practice and handling cases with classical homeopathy. There is a lot of confusion regarding various aspects of clinical practice. 'SHOT' course provides effective solutions to all the queries and removes all the confusion if it exists in a student-physician. Practical topics are covered and case-centered learning sessions are conducted during 'SHOT' orientation course. After completing the course, the student-physician would be in a position to handle various types of cases in clinical practice with greater confidence and ease than he would have otherwise done. 'SHOT' is the first and the most important step in making of a skilled homeopathic physician. The interested physicians can get the details by contacting Dr Deshmukh on email: dradeshmukhin@yahoo.co.in.

The duration of the course is twenty days, which includes lectures and case-centered tutorials. The course also includes sessions on 'How to set up a homoeopathic clinic?' All the students who take admission to 'SHOT' get the benefit of free personality development sessions from the most reputed personality development expert. One can also learn how to build an effective doctor-patient relationship for successful practice

5. HOMOEOPATHIC STUDY CIRCLE

Homoeopathic Study Circle, the oldest and perhaps the first of its kind, is an organisation of homeopathic physicians in central India. Dr S. Karnad and a group of five to six enthusiastic homeopathic physicians of the Nagpur city founded it in the year 1965. The organisation was established with the sole objective of study and propagation of a scientific approach to Hahnemannian Homeopathy. The activities include, lectures on practical topics from Master's of homeopathy, case presentations and study of complicated cases (the case is circulated in advance and case study and active participation of members is sought in the meeting so that the experience is heightened. Physicians have reported that such study of cases allows them to handle even difficult clinical conditions with confidence in their private practice.) Clinical discussions on topic's pertaining to Homeopathic practice are held. Clinical meetings, workshops, and seminars of very high standard are conducted throughout the year. The activities are aimed at establishing norms in prescribing in conformity to the accepted principles of the science. Through its dedicated efforts, this organisation has been able to infuse confidence and incorporate a scientific approach to the homeopathic practice in the physicians as well as the students. HSC is a well-knit family of highly skilled Hahnemannian homeopaths. Being an HSC member itself is a privilege as it immediately brings one in touch with Hahnemannian homeopaths who have been able to translate philosophy into practice. HSC members have the advantage of finding solutions to most complicated problems in day-to-day practice through discussions and exchange of mutual experiences. Members who participate actively in clinical meetings and discussions are awarded with appreciation certificates at the end of each year. For those who have successfully treated cases HSC offers a platform to present their cases, so that others may be benefited from their experience. HSC membership is most beneficial to practitioners who want to excel in homeopathic practice and are willing to acquire new skills every day.

6. DR ROBIN MURPHY, ND

- Dr. Robin Murphy was born on August 15, 1950 in Grand Rapids, Michigan. He carried out his undergraduate studies at the Michigan State University (1972-1976). There he discovered their homoeopathic historical collection and became intrigued with the system and began his studies.

- In 1976 he entered the National College of Naturopathic Medicine (NCNM). There he was awarded the Hahnemann Scholarship for his Thesis: Homoeopathy and Cancer. While at the school he studied with Dr. Ravi Sahni and Dr. John Bastyr. He directed the homoeopathy program at NCNM from 1980-1984. He also taught at Bastyr University.

- He published the Homoeopathic Medical Repertory in 1993 and the Lotus Materia Medica in 1996 which sell like hot cakes even today.
- He is presently the director of the Lotus Medical Centre, located in London, England. LMC sponsors seminars on homoeopathy and oriental medicine throughout the world. The Lotus Medical Centre has educational programs on Qi Medicine and Homoeopathy.

"Murphy was one of the earliest 'seminar' teachers, and is responsible for introducing many people to homoeopathy. His teaching style has been described as 'laid-back' and he brings a clarity to the interrelation between philosophy, materia medica, and repertory work."

Julian Winston
Author of The Faces of Homoeopathy &
The Heritage of Homoeopathic Literature

7. DR FREDERIK SCHROYENS, MD

Dr. Frederik Schroyens, MD, is a 1977 medical graduate of the State University of Ghent (Belgium) and a 1978 graduate of the Homeopathic Training Course at the Faculty for Homeopathy in London (MFHom). In 1981 Schroyens became the president of VSU, the largest homeopathic college in Belgium.

One of the earliest RADAR users in 1986, Schroyens became the homeopathic coordinator of the RADAR project soon afterwards. In 1987 Schroyens was the main link between Vithoulkas and the programming team at the University of Namur during the development of the Vithoulkas Expert System – an algorithm duplicating Vithoulkas' "thought process" which suggests possible remedies for the case at hand.

Culling the homeopathic literature for repertory additions, Schroyens and a team of homeopaths corrected the Kent Repertory, incorporating a number of additions in the RADAR program.

In 1993 Schroyens edited a printed version of Synthesis, the expanded Repertory linked to the RADAR project. A computer version of Synthesis exists in seven languages. Translations into various other languages are ongoing. Since 1995, several books based on Synthesis have been published in several languages, such as 1001 Small Remedies and Arzeimittelbilder vonGemut and Traume.

He published as "Introduction to Homeopathy" in 1984 in Dutch, which has been translated into French and Portuguese.

Dr. Schroyens has been lecturing on homeopathy in most European countries as well as in North and South America. He also has a busy homeopathic practice in Ghent, Belgium.

8. DR ROGER VAN ZANDVOORT

Van Zandvoort was born in Heerlen, Netherlands. After a stint in the army, he went to naturopathic school and became interested in herbalism and later homeopathy. He bought the MacRepertory program in 1987 to help in his practice. He began adding remedies and rubrics to MacRepertory from the common sources – Kent's Materia Medica, Hahnemann's Materia Medical Pura, The Synthetic Repertory of Barthels and Klunker.

David Warkentin saw the work, liked it, and van Zandvoort agreed to publish it. Van Zandvoort now has worked with a team of about 50 people to cull the information needed to produce the Complete Repertory, a massive book.

9. DR LUC DE SCHEPPER, MD

Luc De Schepper, MD, Ph.D., Lic.Ac., is known to hundreds of students as a brilliant and inspiring lecturer and to thousands of patients as a gentle and compassionate healer. Soon after receiving his medical degree in his native Belgium in 1971, he began studying homeopathy as part of a Ph.D. program in acupuncture. He also studied with Robin Murphy and with the British Institute of Homeopathy but learned the most by spending years studying the Old Masters in thousands of old journals. Dr. Luc began incorporating classical homeopathy into his holistic practice upon moving to the US in 1981, using homeopathy exclusively since 1991. His Renaissance Institute of Classical Homeopathy provides professional training in Boston, MA, Secaucus, NJ and Las Vegas, NV to healthcare professionals.

10. DR JEREMY SHERR

Jeremy Sherr was born April 2, 1955, in South Africa, and grew up in Israel.

Homeopathy found him 23 years ago, and Jeremy began formal studies at the College of Homeopathy, London, in 1980. He completed a degree simultaneously in Acupuncture at the International College of Oriental Medicine. Though he has practiced homeopathy exclusively since 1982, his knowledge of Chinese Medicine shines through his homeopathic thinking.

Mr. Sherr began teaching while still in college. He taught in most of the British schools, and began his Dynamis School in 1987. It is the longest running post-graduate course in the UK.

Jeremy has taught the Dynamis curriculum throughout Europe and North America, and is a popular lecturer worldwide. He maintains a busy practice in London, Tel Aviv, and New York.

He was the first to re-develop the science and art of provings after a century of near silence. In 1982 he conducted his first proving of *Scorpion*, and has since completed 21 thorough provings.

He has written *The Dynamics and Methodology of Homeopathic Provings*, which has become a standard textbook in most colleges and the basis of worldwide proving guidelines. It has been translated into French, German, and Russian.

He was awarded a fellowship from the Society of Homeopaths in 1991 and a Ph.D. from Medicina Alternativa. He is a Member of the North American Society of Homeopaths, and is an honorary professor of Yunan Medical College, Kunming, China.

∎

HOMEOPATHY ON INTERNET

A list of some interesting and informative homeopathic websites is given below. Reader can get information about research, clinical training, articles, journals, various national and international organizations and institutions related to homeopathy, online books and useful links on these websites.

www.bjainbooks.com
www.homeopathy.org
www.simillimum.com
www.homeopathic.com
www.alchemilla.com
www.homeopathic.org
www.teleosis.com
www.homeopathyhome.com
www.homeopathyschool.demon.co.uk
www.homeopathytraining.org
www.homeopathyonline.freeserve.co.uk
www.classicalhomeopathy.com
www.homeopathyvancouver.com
www.njhonline.com

BIBLIOGRAPHY

1. Samuel Hahnemann: *Organon of Medicine*, 5th and 6th edition, (B.Jain) *Chronic Diseases, Hahnemann's Lesser Writings* (B.Jain).
2. Von Boenninghausen: *Lesser Writings* (Articles translated from German Journals) (B. Jain).
3. M. L. Dhawale: *Perceiving: 1, Principles and Practice of Homeopathy.*
   Clinical Investigation in Homeopathic Practice, The ICR Operational Manual (ICR).
4. J. T. Kent: *Lesser Writings, Lectures on Homeopathic Philosophy, Lectures on Homeopathic Materia Medica* (B. Jain).
5. R.E. Dudgeon: *Lectures on the Theory & Practice of Homeopathy* (B. Jain).
6. Bernard S. Siegel's article in the 1991 issue of AHHA 'Furthering the Understanding of Holistic Health,' the newsletter of American Holistic Health Association.
7. Stuart Close: *Genius of Homeopathy* (B. Jain).
8. Dr. Joel Kreisberg: Articles *'Homeopathic Education — An Overview'* and *'The Attitude of Homeopathic Education'* on website www.teleosis.com.
9. George Vithoulkas: *The Science of Homeopathy* (B. Jain).
10. Margaret Tyler and Dr. John Weir: *Repertorizing* (B. Jain).
11. Jugal Kishore: *Evolution of Homeopathic Repertories and Repertorization* (B. Jain).

12. P. Sankaran: Collected Writings, *'Elements of Homeopathy'* *'Some Hints on Case Taking'*, 2nd edition, 1968 (Roy &Co.).
13. Shashi Kant Tiwari: *Essentials of Repertorization* (B.Jain).
14. Gustavo Dominici's (Italy): Article *'The Simillimum Route'* in volume 14, 2nd issue of year 2001 of 'Homeopathic Links'.
15. S. M. Gunavante: *Introduction to Homeopathic Prescribing* (B. Jain).
16. I.C.R. Symposium Volumes 'Area D' Perceiving Scientific Method: Repertorization. 'Area G' 'Area H' & 'Area C' (Institute of Clinical Research).
17. I.C.R. Symposium Volume 'Area A'- Philosophical Foundations 'Area B'- Perceiving Mental State and 'Area C'- Perceiving Miasmatic Evolution (ICR).
18. H.A. Roberts: *The Art of Cure by Homeopathy* (B. Jain).
19. Rajan Sankaran: *'Spirit of Homeopathy'*.
20. David Little: www.simillimum.com –The online library.
21. Jeremy Sherr: Article *'Medicine of the Future'* magazine—The Homeopathic Heritage, Volume 27, December, 2002.
22. Fons Vanden Berghe, (Belgium): Article *'Clinical Training in Classical Homeopathy'* magazine—Homeopathic Links, Volume II, 2/98.
23. Helmut Sydow: *Learning Classical Homeopathy* (B. Jain).
24. Will Taylor, MD 1998: *'The Development of Dose and Potency in the History of Homeopathy'*.
25. Elizabeth Wright-Hubbard: *A Brief Study Course in Homeopathy*.
26. Dr. Proceso Sanchez Ortgea: *Notes on the Miasms* (English Edition) 1980 (National Homeopathic Pharmacy, New Delhi).
27. S.C. Basu: *Handbook of Preventive and Social Medicine*, 2nd edition, 1991 (Current Books International, Calcutta).

28. Steven A. Harold: *Marketing for Complementary Therapists* (B. Jain).
29. Michael Swash: *Hutchison's Clinical Methods,* Nineteenth Edition, (ELBS).
30. Dr. K.N. Kasad: 'Area G' (G.2) I.C.R. Symposium Volumes, *'Homeopathic Prescribing: Acute-Chronic'.*

    'The Unbalanced Image: Standardized Programming' (ICR).
31. Rachel Webb: *Article on Decorating Home Offices* (internet website Pagewise.com) (Pagewise, Inc.).
32. Pierre Schmidt: The Homeopathic Consultation *'The Art of Interrogation'* (B. Jain).
33. Margaret Tyler: *How not to do it* (B. Jain).
34. D. Tarafdar: *Repertory Explained,* 2nd edition, 1993 (Modern Homeopathic Publication).
35. Ramanlal P. Patel: *The Art of Case-taking & Practical Repertorization in Homeopathy,* 6th edition, 1998 (Sai Homeopathic Book Corporation, Kottayam).